Wheezing Disorders in the Preschool Child

Pathophysiology and Management

Wheezing Disorders in the Preschool Child

Pathophysiology and Management

Fernando Martinez MD
Swift-McNear Professor of Pediatrics
Director, Arizona Respiratory Center
University of Arizona
Tucson AZ
USA

Simon Godfrey MD, PhD, FRCP
Professor of Pediatrics
Director, Institute of Pulmonology
Hadassah University Hospital
Jerusalem
Israel

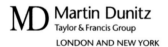
Martin Dunitz
Taylor & Francis Group
LONDON AND NEW YORK

© 2003 Martin Dunitz, an imprint of the Taylor & Francis Group plc

First published in 2003
Published in the USA and Canada by
Martin Dunitz, Taylor & Francis Group
29 West 35th Street, New York, NY 10001
and in the UK by
Martin Dunitz, Taylor & Francis Group plc
11 New Fetter Lane, London EC4P 4EE

Website: http://www.dunitz.co.uk

Although every effort has been made to ensure that all owners of copyright material have been acknowledged in this publication, we would be glad to acknowledge in subsequent reprints or editions any omissions brought to our attention.

A CIP record for this book is available from the British Library.

ISBN 1 84184 155 2

Distributed in the USA by
Fulfilment Center
Taylor & Francis
10650 Toebben Drive
Independence, KY 41051, USA
Toll Free Tel.: +1 800 634 7064
E-mail: taylorandfrancis@thomsonlearning.com

Distributed in Canada by
Taylor & Francis
74 Rolark Drive
Scarborough, Ontario M1R 4G2, Canada
Toll Free Tel.: +1 877 226 2237
E-mail: tal_fran@istar.ca

Distributed in the rest of the world by
Thomson Publishing Services
Cheriton House
North Way
Andover, Hampshire SP10 5BE, UK
Tel.: +44 (0)1264 332424
E-mail: salesorder.tandf@thomsonpublishingservices.co.uk

Composition by EXPO Holdings, Petaling Jaya, Malaysia

Printed and bound in Spain by Grafos, S.A.

Contents

Preface

One of the most common and yet most challenging problems facing the pediatrician is the nature and management of the wheezy infant and preschool child. In some countries, such as the USA and Australia, the incidence of wheezing can reach up to 50%. Although the incidence is rather less in Europe, the wheezy infant and preschool child still occupies a very large part of the time of the pediatrician and constitutes a considerable burden on the delivery of health care. The parents of the wheezy infant or preschool child are naturally worried about what is the matter with their child, how the child should be treated and what is the long-term prognosis. 'Will he/she have asthma all his/her life, doctor?' must surely be one of the most frequent questions posed to the pediatrician caring for young children. It is little comfort to the parents, or indeed to the pediatrician, when we admit that we are not sure about the cause of the wheezing and even less sure about the correct management, if we are honest, in this era of evidence-based medicine.

This lack of knowledge about wheezing in early life is perplexing, given the large amount of resources that have been dedicated to research about the pathogenesis and treatment of asthma during the past decades. There is little doubt that these efforts have produced medicines that, when used appropriately, allow 90% of school children and adults with asthma to lead a perfectly normal life. It is also evident, however, that there is no way to prevent the development of chronic asthma and that many patients with asthma require continued controller treatment for years. As will be discussed in several chapters of this book, one of the intriguing recent findings from longitudinal studies of asthma is that, in most severe cases of the disease, the first asthma-like symptoms occur during the preschool years. If a strategy for the primary prevention of asthma will ever be successful, we will need to understand much better which factors determine the initiation of the most severe forms of the disease during the first years of life.

In view of the challenges posed by the wheezy infant and preschool child, both for the clinician and the interested researcher, we decided to collaborate on this book in order to collect and collate as much objective information as possible and present it to the reader in a manner which will at least lead to a better familiarity with the condition. We chose to work together rather than to produce a large multi-author book because we wanted to present the reader with the information in a logical and readable fashion with the practicing clinician in mind. Between us we have considerable experience in the clinical, epidemiologic and physiologic aspects of the wheezy infant and preschool child, and each chapter represents a joint effort. Despite our desire to produce a book suitable for the clinician, we have not neglected the basic science aspects of the problem and we have included extensive referencing to published works with which we are familiar so that the clinical or basic scientist can refer back to evaluate the original data. We have limited ourselves very strictly to the preschool years – approximately from birth to 5 or 6 years of age – because this is the period, especially in the first three years of life, when wheezing is most difficult to evaluate and manage. We did not intend to write about asthma in older children, which presents much less of a diagnostic and management problem and for which there are already many excellent texts. Because of the pivotal role of viral infection, especially infection by the respiratory syncytial virus, in causing infants and young children to wheeze, we have devoted a chapter to this specific cause of wheezing and its management.

Why, then, is there the need for a book such as this and why does wheezing in early childhood present such difficulties? Perhaps the most pressing reason is that there are many causes of wheezing in this age group but to all intents and purposes the clinical presentation is very similar or even identical. Moreover, the clinical findings and diagnostic tests available at the present time rarely give a conclusive answer as to the nature of the problem in what we shall be calling the typical wheezy infant or preschool child, i.e. those with no specific disease causing the wheezing. Parents, however intelligent and well meaning, often find it very difficult to describe the nature of the noisy breathing or respiratory distress from which their child suffers and this is particularly problematic since the child may well be completely asymptomatic by the time he/she reaches the doctor's office. During an attack the typical wheezy infant or preschool child will be distressed with generalized, musical wheezing, hyperinflation and a normal chest radiograph, whatever the origin of the wheeze. However, an almost identical picture can be due to such important and potentially dangerous atypical causes of wheezing such as gastroesophageal reflux, cystic fibrosis, primary ciliary dyskinesia and congenital anomalies of the airways, lungs or heart. The measurement of lung function or bronchial responsivity can often help with the evaluation of the older wheezy child or adult, but lung function testing in infants or very young children is not readily available and is confined to very specialized centers. Even in these centers, the role of lung function testing in the management of most wheezy infants or preschool children is far from clear. The management of the primary disease obviously determines the management of the atypical wheezy infant with a specific diagnosis such as cystic fibrosis. With the typical wheezy infant, in whom there is no other underlying disease, suggestions for management are very confusing. Some published asthma management guidelines recommend treatment of the wheezy infant as if they were all little asthmatics in terms of evaluation and management with absolutely no evidence to support this approach, nor, in many instances, any hope of carrying it out. But parents expect us to be able to help their wheezy child and are rarely willing to sit by and watch the child without doing anything therapeutically meaningful. In this book we suggest what we believe to be a simple, logical and safe approach to management based on trial and error, which also ensures that children should not continue to receive treatment which is ineffective.

The epidemiology and immunology of the typical wheezy infant and preschool child provides some clues as to the nature of the conditions causing wheezing in this age group and we have paid particular attention to these aspects of the problem. For some years, we and others have been aware that there are at least three main groups of infants who wheeze in early childhood: (1) those with rather narrow airways to begin with, (2) those who wheeze in response to viral infections and (3) those with a strong atopic background. We discuss these types of wheezy children and consider what is known about the induction of wheezing, its course and the long-term prognosis. Recent epidemiologic studies have begun to shed considerable light on the way environmental factors may influence the developing immune system of the infant in such a way as to predispose or inhibit the child from becoming wheezy or developing allergic diseases. Some of this evidence is confusing and even contradictory, and we have paid particular attention to presenting a fair and balanced account of this fascinating and developing story. Throughout the book we report what we really do and do not know, and in the last chapter we present a wish list of suggestions as to what might be done to further clarify the nature and management of wheezing in infancy and early childhood.

Finally, we wish to express our sincere appreciation of the help we have received from our publishers. In particular, we thank Martin Dunitz himself for his encouragement and practical support which enabled us to collaborate so easily over a distance of some 9000 miles. Peter Stevenson was the managing editor of this project and we are especially grateful to him for his friendship, help and patience throughout.

Fernando Martinez
Simon Godfrey

1
Epidemiology of wheezing in infants and preschool children

The past decade has witnessed significant advances in our understanding of the epidemiology of wheezing illnesses occurring during the first years of life. Several longitudinal studies initiated either during pregnancy or at birth, and in which follow-up has been extended beyond the preschool years, have provided a new perspective on the risk factors for and prognosis of these illnesses. There is now clear evidence indicating that wheezing in early life is a heterogeneous condition, in which recurrent episodes of airway obstruction are the final common pathway for the expression of different underlying mechanisms and, ultimately, for different diseases. This marked heterogeneity may explain the difficulty that most clinicians encounter in treating these illnesses which appear to be less responsive to the usually successful treatment prescribed to older children and adults with asthma (see Chapter 7). There are also 'atypical' forms of noisy breathing in this age group that contribute to the complexity of their diagnosis and treatment (see Chapter 4). However, even when confronted with the typical presentation of this condition the pediatrician is often unable to predict the response to therapy and to answer the most pressing question of parents, 'Does my child have asthma?'. In this review of the epidemiology of wheezing diseases in early life an attempt will be made to provide a logical basis to explain the nature of the problem.

INCIDENCE OF FIRST EPISODES OF WHEEZING

In epidemiological terms, incidence is the number of new cases of a certain condition that occur in a population in a given unit of time. It needs to be distinguished from prevalence, which is the proportion of all subjects in a population who have a certain condition at any given time. In this section, incidence of wheezing, regardless of the mechanism involved, will be described. Incidence and prevalence of different forms of wheezing will be assessed in the section dedicated to each of these forms.

Wheezing is a very uncommon clinical finding during the first 1–2 months of life.[1] Why neonates are spared from the clinical manifestations of airway obstruction is not understood. Since most wheezing lower respiratory illnesses (LRI) in this age group are associated with viral infection (see below), it is plausible to surmise that maternal or developmental factors may determine a different immune response to viruses in the neonate. However, the data favoring such an assumption are scanty. It has also been suggested that the structure of the lung during this period of life may protect neonates

1

against severe airway obstruction,[2] but the lack of solid anatomic data precludes definitive conclusions. The fact remains, however, that apnea and not wheezing is the most
common manifestation of respiratory syncytial virus (RSV) infection before 2 months
of age.

After 2 months of age, incidence of first episodes of wheezing increase markedly,
reaching a peak between 2 and 5 months of age.[3] Incidence decreases after the sixth
month of life, and remains low and relatively stable during the second and third years of
life.[4] There is no clear explanation for this very consistent pattern for the timing of the
first wheezing episodes. It is possible that it is simply a probabilistic distribution of
events that occur after the refractory newborn period. It is also possible that airway
growth may lag somatic growth during a 4–5-month period in which weight is doubling
and length is increasing by 25%. This may explain why a recent analysis of maximal
expiratory flows obtained with the chest compression technique showed a curvilinear
pattern, with growth of flows becoming faster after 6 months of age, particularly in
males.[5] In other words, maximal expiratory flow lags somatic growth for the first few
months of life. The maturation of immune responses in the post-neonatal period may
also increase the risk of developing airway inflammation during viral infections.[3]

INFECTION AS A FACTOR IN THE ETIOLOGY OF WHEEZING

Several studies have demonstrated that most episodes of wheezing (be it first episode or
subsequent recurrence) during the first three years of life are associated with evidence
of viral infection.[4,6,7] Until recently, the most frequent viruses isolated from nasopharyngeal samples (either by immunofluorescence or culture) or detected by shifts in
specific immunoglobulin serum titers were RSV, parainfluenza and adenoviruses.[7] Up to
80% of all incident episodes of wheezing were thought to be due to infections by these
viruses. In rare cases, influenza viruses, *Chlamydia tracomatis* or *Chlamydia pneumonia*,
and *Mycoplasma pneumonia*, had been isolated during wheezing episodes in this age
group.[8] For years, the predominant belief was that rhinoviruses (RV) were rarely associated with upper or lower respiratory illnesses before the age of 3.[4] However, RV are
difficult to isolate with traditional virological techniques requiring antibodies because of
their great genomic variability, giving rise to more than 100 serotypes. The availability
of molecular biology techniques using reverse-transcriptase-polymerase chain reaction
(PCR) has provided a completely new perspective regarding the etiology of wheezing in
early life.[9] It has now been reported that RV can be isolated in approximately a quarter
of all infants hospitalized with a diagnosis of LRI during the first year of life, all of
whom were wheezing on admission.[10,11] This makes RV the second most frequently isolated virus during wheezing LRI in this age group. In many of these infants, RV isolation occurred in concomitance with detection of RSV, and the great majority of multiple
virus infections were due to the RSV/RV combination. In one study, results suggested
that RV identification was associated with increased severity of bronchiolitis,[10] but over
half of all patients with RV had more than one virus detected. Therefore, the independent role of RV in determining disease severity could not be distinguished from that of
RV as a co-adjuvant of RSV infection. Nevertheless, these new data on the role of RV in

early wheezing suggest that the proportion of first episodes of wheezing due to viral infection may far exceed 80% and more likely close to 100%.

Older studies had suggested that viral isolation during wheezing LRI decreased markedly during the second and third years of life as compared to the very high frequency of isolation during the first year. In fact, viruses could be detected in only 40–50% of 2-year-old children with acute wheezing LRI (Children's Respiratory Study, unpublished observations). It is likely that this conclusion will need to be revisited, in view of the very large proportion of infants in whom RV has been recently detected even during the first year of life. Further studies will certainly add valuable information to this field in the near future.

Advances in microbiology have also suggested that other heretofore unknown organisms may play a role in LRI in early life. A new member of the paramyxovirus family from the *Metapneumovirus* genus was recently isolated, a genus in which only avian viruses had been described.[12] Children in whom this virus was isolated had clinical symptoms that strikingly resembled those associated with RSV. Interestingly, serologic studies showed that, much like for RSV, almost all children are infected by human *Metapneumovirus* by the age of 5, and that the virus has been infecting humans at least for the past 50 years. No comprehensive epidemiological studies have addressed the public health impact and the incidence of infection due to this virus in large population samples. Nevertheless, a preliminary report from Australia suggested that metapneumoviruses may cause wheezing LRI in a small fraction of infants and young children.[13]

RECURRENCE OF WHEEZING AND ITS CAUSES

One of the most striking epidemiological characteristics of wheezing episodes in infants and young children is their tendency to recur. Although many children in this age group can have a single episode of wheezing not followed by subsequent similar episodes, no less than 50% of such subjects will present with wheezing at least once within the next few months. Moreover, parents of 30–40% of children who wheeze before the age of 3 report current wheezing at 6 years of age.[14,15] This type of presentation thus suggests two potential scenarios: either recurrent wheezing is the result of underlying predisposing factors that explain both initial and subsequent episodes, or the initial episode creates the conditions for changes in the host that predispose her/him to subsequent similar symptoms.

In order to understand better what determines recurrent wheezing, several groups of investigators have followed infants and young children with this condition and have assessed risk factors and long-term outcomes of these subjects. Results from these studies have suggested that recurrent wheezing is a heterogeneous condition and that different recurrent wheezing phenotypes coexist in this age group. This has been a rather unexpected finding because the clinical presentation of infants with recurrent wheezing does not provide clues to the clinician that would suggest the existence of different subgroups of subjects. Nevertheless, the appreciation that recurrent early childhood wheezing is not a single entity has helped clinicians and caregivers, both of whom need to provide answers to pressing questions from concerned parents regarding the prognosis of this condition in their children. In addition, this new knowledge has suggested new avenues for the primary and secondary prevention of asthma and asthma-like conditions, as will be discussed in Chapter 8.

What follows is a description of the three most common recurrent wheezing phenotypes that have been identified in epidemiological studies. It is important to understand that there may be overlap between these different conditions, simply because it is not always possible to identify absolute thresholds for complex risk factors and, therefore, no marker perfectly distinguishes between the different phenotypes described herein. However, in spite of the many gray areas, efforts are currently under way to better understand the different risk factors that predominate in one phenotype or the other. The classification described below is also different from the three subdivisions of wheezing in the first three years of life reported earlier by Martinez et al[14] – transient wheezers, late-onset wheezers and persistent wheezers. The first group is still included in the new classification, but new data and insights obtained after the publication of that study have driven us to conclude that although the timing of initiation of symptoms is very important, more significant in terms of long-term prognosis, risk factors and immunopathogenesis is the distinction between non-atopic and atopic forms of wheezing. Both late-onset and persistent wheezing can be atopic and non-atopic (Figure 1.1), and the potential role of late or early initiation of symptoms will be discussed separately for each form below.

Transient early wheezing (60% of wheezers < 3 years of age)

The existence of a group of infants and young children who present with recurrent wheezing episodes during the first year of life and show apparent remission of these

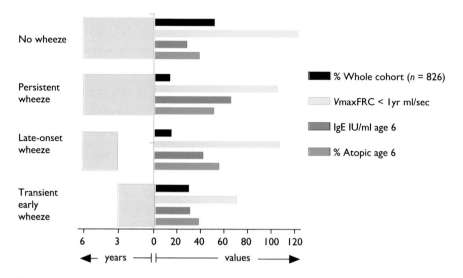

Figure 1.1

Asthma and wheezing in the first six years of life (from Martinez et al[14]).

symptoms by the early school years has been known for a long time.[16,17] However, a more thorough identification of this phenotype has only become available more recently, the result of longitudinal studies starting at birth. These studies have demonstrated that no less than 60% of all wheezing babies and young children have stopped all wheezing by 3–6 years of age. These children are not more likely to have a family history of asthma or to have personal or family history of allergic conditions such as eczema or skin-test reactivity to allergens than children who do not wheeze during the first six years of life.[14,18] Symptoms usually begin during the first year of life and may either subside or continue into the second and third years of life.[15] Although longitudinal studies have shown that children belonging to this group tend to have symptoms almost exclusively during viral infections, the severity of each of these episodes does not appear to be less prominent in this particular group as compared with those observed in persistent wheezers. This is important from a clinical point of view because transient early wheezers cannot be identified with those young children who in the past were called 'happy wheezers'. Moreover, studies in older atopic wheezers have demonstrated that the severity of symptoms during the early school years is a very important predictor of subsequent persistence and severity of wheezing. However, this does not hold true for wheezing during the first years of life. It is very important for the clinician to understand these differences in the natural history of recurrent wheezing at different ages because prognosis is an important concern for parents, and labeling an infant or preschool child as having asthma (with its associated stigma of a lifelong, chronic disease) simply because her/his symptoms are quite severe may be misguided in this age group.

Risk factors for transient early wheezing

Infants of mothers who smoke during pregnancy are much more likely to have transient wheezing episodes during the first years of life.[19] This is one of the most consistent findings in all pediatric epidemiologic studies.[20]

Another factor that seems to be strongly associated with transient infant wheezing is the level of lung function measured shortly after birth and before any wheezing episode occurs.[21,22] The consistency of this finding in many epidemiologic studies suggests that either a functional or structural alteration of the lung is present in many of the children that predisposes them to wheezing. This makes physiologic sense because resistance to the flow of a gas through a tube is proportional to the fourth power of the radius. Thus, it is plausible to suggest that in airways with a smaller initial diameter, larger increases in resistance will occur with the same amount of airway mucus or edema during a viral infection. In favor of the hypothesis that this may be a structural alteration are studies showing that transient infant wheezers did not have an increased prevalence of methacholine hyperresponsiveness or positive peak flow variability at 11 years of age.[23] This, in spite of the fact that levels of lung function, especially indices related to forced expiratory flows at low lung volumes, were significantly lower in transient infant wheezers both at 11 and 16 years of age.

It is interesting to stress here that when lung function measured shortly after birth was compared in different groups of wheezing infants and young children, only those who would be later classified as transient wheezers showed diminished maximal expiratory flows. These results suggest that persistent wheezers do not start life with an altered lung function but acquire these alterations postnatally. This issue will be discussed in more detail later in this chapter. However, it is reasonable to surmise that if children with diminished lung function at birth are also at risk for atopic wheezing then they are more likely to have increased severity of wheezing in early life and increased likelihood of persistence of symptoms thereafter.

Environmental exposures also seem to play an important role as risk factors for transient infant wheezing. Children who attend daycare during the first months of life or who live with older siblings at home are more likely to wheeze in early life, but this increased risk does not seem to extend beyond the age of 4–6.[24] Exposure to increased levels of house dust endotoxin has also been shown to be associated with increased risk of wheezing during the first years of life, but this risk does not seem to extend beyond the first three to six years of life either.[25] Moreover, endotoxin exposure in early life appears to decrease the risk of subsequent development of atopic wheezing and allergic sensitization during the school years. This apparent contradiction is discussed in more detail in Chapter 3. Exposure to allergens such as cockroaches[26] is also associated with significant increased risk of wheezing during the first years of life, without concomitant increased risk of developing allergic sensitization to these or other allergens before the age of 3. It is therefore possible that factors that increase irritation of the airways or upregulate immune responses to viruses may increase the incidence of transient wheezing in early life, but this issue requires further elucidation.

Male sex is also very strongly associated with the risk of transient infant wheezing.[15,18] This finding is of great interest because a recent, very large, multicenter analysis of lung function during the first year of life confirmed that girls have larger size-corrected maximal expiratory flows obtained with the chest compression technique than males.[5] The hypothesis that airway structure may be an important determinant factor for transient infant wheezing is supported by this correspondence between levels of lung function, gender and risk for this condition.

An intriguing finding of three longitudinal studies[15,18,27] is that children of younger mothers are more likely to have transient infant wheezing than children of older mothers. There is no clear explanation for this finding but children of younger mothers are also of a lower birthweight than those of older mothers.[27] It is thus possible that, much like for somatic growth, airway growth may also be related to maternal age. There indeed appears to be some evidence that children of younger mothers have lower levels of lung function than those of older mothers.[27]

Finally, bottle-feeding is also associated with transient infant wheezing.[15,18,28] The mechanisms by which breastfeeding may decrease the risk of transient infant wheezing may have to do with protection against the development of more severe viral infections. The protective effect of breastfeeding disappears with age and is not observed for persistent wheezing.

Non-atopic persistent wheezing (20% of wheezers < 3 years of age)

As explained earlier, approximately 40% of all children who wheeze during the first three years of life have parental reports of continued wheezing at the age of 6.

Only about half of these persistent wheezers have evidence of sensitization against local aeroallergens, which contrasts with > 90% of allergic children among those who have current wheezing at age 13.[29] For years, the issue remained unresolved as to whether these non-atopic wheezers of the toddler and early school years were to become the future allergic asthmatics or if these children were a different phenotype of childhood wheezing. This is certainly not an academic matter because it is a common belief among experienced pediatricians and specialists that toddlers do not respond as well as older children to the most widely used anti-inflammatory and bronchodilator therapies successfully used in older children and adults with asthma. Moreover, many children presenting with wheezing in this age group have symptoms mainly during the winter months, a time when viral infections are most prevalent in the community. It was thus suspected, but never substantiated in controlled studies, that there was a group of preschoolers who had airway obstruction mainly during viral infections, that their symptoms, much like those of transient wheezers, were not associated with increased prevalence of allergic sensitization and that their prognosis was better than that of atopic wheezers.

Recent longitudinal studies have confirmed this suspicion. When preschool wheezers were followed up to the school years, it was found that by early adolescence most of those who were non-atopic were no longer wheezing.[30] The main factor associated with this form of wheezing was the age at which their wheezing had started: the majority of these children had objective evidence of wheezing LRI during the first year of life, whereas those with atopy-associated wheezing were more often reported to have their first wheezing episodes during the second or third years of life. This pattern of presentation of non-atopic wheezing was confirmed when the data were analyzed in a different way: the outcome up to the age of 13 of the first episode of LRI occurring before 3 years of age was assessed prospectively according to its etiology.[31] A consistent pattern was observed for children who had confirmed RSV-LRI, most of these occurring during the first year of life as described earlier: these children were three to four times more likely to wheeze at the age of 6 than their peers without RSV-LRI. However, this increased risk withered markedly with age and the risk of wheezing in children with RSV-LRI was only marginally increased by the age of 13. Children with confirmed RSV-LRI were not more likely to be atopic or to have elevated serum IgE levels at the age of 11. Thus, both retrospective and prospective analysis of the data gave the same result: a group of children, most of whom wheezed during RSV infection in early life, were more likely to wheeze, especially during the toddler years, and this form of wheezing was unrelated to allergic sensitization. The natural trend of this form of wheezing was to remit with age, and thus the decreasing association between RSV-LRI and wheezing between the ages of 6 and 13.

Although in studies performed in developed English-speaking countries non-atopic wheezers are already a minority among children who wheeze during the early school years, the same does not appear to hold true in all populations and in all latitudes. Likewise, empirical observations suggest that the generally good long-term prognosis of non-atopic wheezing in toddlers raised in developed societies may not be observed in underdeveloped countries. Recent studies from Australia, Peru and Ethiopia illustrate this point. In Australia, comparisons of the prevalence of asthma symptoms and atopy were made between Aboriginal and non-Aboriginal children between the ages of 7 and 12 living in the same rural communities.[32] As a group, Aboriginal children were significantly less likely to be atopic and to have allergic rhinitis than non-Aboriginal children, but were equally likely to wheeze (31.0 versus 27.3%) and to have a diagnosis of asthma (39.4 versus 39.3%). Among Aboriginal children, having had bronchitis before the age of 2 was a strong risk factor for wheeze (adjusted odds ratio of 9.3) and asthma (adjusted odds ratio of 19.3). This contrasted with what was observed in Caucasian children in whom, much like in the Tucson study described earlier, bronchitis before the age of 2 was only weakly associated with current asthma and wheezing between the ages of 7 and 12. In the Peruvian study, 8–10-year-old children living in a deprived urban area of Lima were studied.[33] Those with reported wheezing during the previous year had mild symptoms and were not more likely to be atopic than those without wheezing, but they did have diminished levels of lung function and were more likely to have exercise-induced falls in lung function. Finally, in Ethiopia, schoolchildren living in rural areas who wheezed were not more likely to be atopic than those who did not wheeze, whereas those living in urban areas showed a significant association between asthma symptoms and allergic sensitization.[34] Therefore, the natural history and prognosis of non-atopic wheezing differs by socioeconomic status of the population, by environmental exposures, by ethnic group and likely by genetic background. Certainly, increased exposure to viral infection in children of lower socioeconomic status increases the likelihood of viral-associated wheezing. But the increased prevalence of non-atopic wheezing relative to atopic wheezing must also be due to a decreased likelihood of the form of allergic sensitization which is characteristic of atopic wheezing among children living in rural areas or in deprived social conditions. It is possible that increased exposure to microbes in general, which is characteristic of small children living in poverty, may have a dual effect. On the one hand, it would be associated with an increase in the incidence of viral and bacterial infection, with consequent more severe airway damage and persistence of wheezing associated with viral infection into the late school years. On the other hand, the same infections that increase the risk of non-atopic persistent wheezing in susceptible individuals may decrease the likelihood of allergic sensitization and of atopic wheezing, the mechanisms of which will be explained in greater detail in Chapter 3.

Risk factors for non-atopic persistent wheezing

We are only beginning to understand what determines non-atopic wheezing in toddlers and schoolchildren. The suspicion that functional characteristics of the lung are involved was suggested many years ago when it was found that children with a history of RSV-LRI had lower levels of lung function and increased prevalence of bronchial hyperresponsiveness (BHR) during the school years than those without such a history.[35,36] This hypothesis was confirmed by two recent longitudinal studies. Data from the Tucson Children's Respiratory Study showed that those with a history of RSV-LRI have diminished lung function at the age of 11, independent of current wheezing at that age.[31] However, a history of RSV-LRI was also associated with marked increase responses to a bronchodilator.[31] As a consequence, post-bronchodilator lung function was not significantly different between children with and without a history of RSV-LRI.

These data, together with findings from the Peruvian study quoted earlier, suggest that RSV-LRI, and perhaps subsequent non-atopic wheezing, is due to an alteration in the regulation of airway tone which makes children more likely to wheeze during viral infections.

What determines this alteration is not known. Two main scenarios are possible: either the increased airway lability observed in these children is genetically determined and is thus present before these children develop the condition; or it is the consequence of damage inflicted to the airways by the initial episode due to RSV or by the subsequent recurrence of viral infections. A third scenario would combine these two: significant airway damage and alteration in the regulation of airway tone could occur in genetically susceptible children during viral infections. A longitudinal study from Australia (this time, among Caucasian children) suggests that the alterations in airway tone observed among non-atopic wheezers may be, at least in part, genetic or congenital. In this study, BHR was assessed in infants shortly after birth by use of the chest compression technique before and after inhalation of histamine.[37] Children were then followed up to the age of 6, when they were assessed for symptoms, allergy skin-test reactivity and again for BHR to histamine, now using voluntary maneuvers. There was no association between BHR at birth and baseline lung function at that same age, nor was there any association between BHR at birth and at 6 years of age. However, there was a significant association between BHR at birth and both wheezing and lung function at the age of 6, and this was independent of atopy at that same age. Moreover, BHR at the age of 6 was also strongly associated with wheezing at that same age, with both forms of BHR (congenital and at the age of 6) contributing separately to the risk of wheezing at the age of 6. Although follow-up at the age of 11 is not yet available for this population, one can speculate that BHR at birth is measuring a genetic characteristic of the airways that may predispose to non-atopic wheezing which is independent of allergic sensitization. Conversely, BHR at the age of 6 is also determined by the atopic status of the child. These two differential determinants of BHR, one related to some intrinsic characteristic of the lung and airways and the other acquired as a consequence of 'lung remodeling', are physiologically plausible and have been described in animal models of asthma.[38] Because the congenital form is most likely structural and thus purportedly unrelated to lung inflammation, one would expect it to be less responsive to inhaled corticosteroids. Unfortunately, no studies have systematically attempted to assess differential responsiveness to anti-inflammatory medication in children with atopic non-atopic wheezing.

The results of the studies described above do not rule out the possibility that alterations in the regulation of airway tone may occur as a consequence of viral infection in susceptible children. Animal models, for example, suggest that infection with RSV in young animals may cause prolonged alterations in airway structure and function.[39] In humans, the prolonged sequelae observed in subjects with bronchiolitis obliterans, caused by infection with certain strains of adenovirus in susceptible infants, constitute a 'proof of concept' for the idea that viruses can indeed cause long-term lung and airway damage. Unfortunately, longitudinal studies in which RSV and other common respiratory viruses have been shown to produce similar (albeit less severe) airway damage are not available.

A special group of non-atopic wheezers that deserves consideration in the framework of this discussion are premature children. Children born before term are more likely to wheeze later in life than their peers born at term.[40] There is a dose–response relation between duration of pregnancy and likelihood of wheezing: every extra week of gestation reduces the risk of severe wheeze during childhood by about 10%. This increased risk does not seem to persist beyond childhood: conscripts born prematurely are not more likely to report current asthma than those born at term.[41] It is now also well established that not only are children born prematurely not more likely to be atopic, but they may even be less likely to have positive skin-test reactivity to allergens and less likely to have eczema than term children.[42] What causes non-atopic wheezing in former 'premies' is still to be determined. Prematurely born children of school age have significantly lower levels of lung function and increased BHR, regardless of their history of bronchopulmonary dysplasia.[43] Clinical trials, albeit with small numbers of subjects, have failed to show that this form of non-atopic wheezing is responsive to treatment with inhaled corticosteroids.[44,45] It is thus possible that premature birth may be associated with BHR that is unrelated to the type of airway inflammation that is characteristic of atopic asthma. It is tempting to speculate that the alterations in airway tone and lung function present in these children are similar to those of other forms of non-atopic wheezing, but there are no solid data to support this speculation. Premature children show marked responses to bronchodilators,[46] much like other non-atopic wheezers do. In one potential scenario, this alteration in the control of airway tone may be present at birth and be a marker of altered autonomous regulation that explains both prematurity and increased risk of wheezing. It is also possible that BHR may be the consequence of early birth, perhaps due to a disruption in the developmental program of lung and airways.

Determinants of the natural history of non-atopic wheezing

The concept that non-atopic wheezing is caused by alterations in the regulation of airway tone not caused by allergies provides clues as to what may explain the tendency for the prevalence of this condition to decrease with age. Results of a longitudinal study of changes in BHR with age performed in Dunedin, New Zealand, shed light on this matter. In this study, a group of almost 1000 children enrolled at birth were challenged with methacholine at 9, 11, 13 and 15 years of age. Skin-test reactivity to allergens and prevalence of wheezing were also assessed at different ages. The authors found that prevalence of methacholine BHR decreased significantly with age, but only among children with either low levels of circulating immunoglobulin E (IgE) or those who were not sensitized against local aeroallergens.[47] Conversely, among children who were skin-test positive, prevalence of methacholine BHR remained high and did not decrease with age. By the age of 13, much like in the Tucson study, all children with a diagnosis of current asthma and who had methacholine BHR were atopic. These results suggest that the form of BHR that is unrelated to atopy tends to decrease with age concomitantly with the marked decrease in the prevalence of non-atopic wheezing. Although not definite, these studies strongly suggest that the physiological decrease in non-atopic BHR that occurs during the school years is an important determinant of the natural tendency for non-atopic wheezing to decrease with age. What determines this age-related decrease in non-atopic BHR is not known. It is possible that lung and airway growth may induce changes in the geometry of the airways and this in turn may cause decreases in BHR. These issues require further longitudinal studies.

Atopic wheezing (20% of wheezers < 3 years of age)

Although atopic asthma of the school years and adult life can start at any age, most cases have their first symptoms during the first six years of life. This remarkable finding has marked recent studies of the natural history of asthma. Therefore, children who are destined to be the future persistent asthmatics intermingle with transient wheezers and non-atopic wheezers during infancy and the toddler years. The immune factors that determine the initiation of atopic asthma and their interaction with relevant environmental stimuli will be addressed elsewhere (see Chapter 3). Here we will review the risk factors for and prognosis of atopic wheezing.

Risk factors for atopic wheezing

Atopy and atopic wheezing

As stated earlier, the future atopic wheezers cannot be distinguished clinically from other wheezing children during the first three years of life, but wheezing usually starts later in this group than in other young wheezers, perhaps more often during the second and third years of life. Although symptoms tend to be more severe in atopic wheezers than in other groups, and they may occur both with and without colds, there is considerable overlap between groups, and the clinician has no single sign, symptom or even laboratory analysis or combination thereof that will allow her/him to recognize atopic wheezers. However, a careful history could be very helpful. When compared with other groups, atopic wheezers are four times more likely to have a family history of asthma and two to three times more likely to have a history of atopic dermatitis than other wheezing groups in this age range. Only a minority of infants who will eventually be classified as atopic wheezers show positive skin-test reactivity against local aeroallergens, to which all will eventually become sensitized later in life.[46] In fact, the prevalence of detectable circulating specific IgE against such aeroallergens in the population as a whole is very low. However, the few infants in whom specific IgE against aeroallergens is detectable in serum are almost invariably destined to wheeze later in life, regardless of whether they have wheezing episodes in the first years of life (most do). This creates a paradoxical situation: not all infants (not even a majority of them) who will go on to be classified as atopic wheezers are atopic (i.e. skin-test positive to aeroallergens) at the time of their initial wheezing episodes. In most, IgE against the most common aeroallergens present in their community will only become detectable months or years after these first episodes. This seriously challenges the hypothesis that the development of specific IgE against aeroallergens 'causes' asthma in these children (this issue will be addressed in more detail in Chapter 3). However, one further piece of evidence coming from the epidemiological literature offers some important clues: children who are sensitized against food antigens in early life and who also become sensitized against aeroallergens by the age of 7 are more likely to have asthma at that age than those who are sensitized against aeroallergens by 7 years of age but who were not sensitized against foods in early life.[48] Conversely, children who are sensitized against food antigens in early life but who do not develop specific IgE against aeroallergens by the age of 7 are not more likely to wheeze at this latter age than those who are not sensitized at either age. Most children who are sensitized against food antigens in early life show no evidence that they are still producing IgE against such antigens by the early school years. In addition, and apart from anecdotal reports, there is no consistent evidence suggesting that exposure to food allergens causes airway obstruction in infants who are sensitized against such allergens. It is thus not plausible to conclude from these data that children with early sensitization against foods who later 'switch' to aeroallergens first have symptoms due to food allergy and later have symptoms attributable to aeroallergens. More likely, the demonstration of positive IgE responses to food antigens in early life in future atopic wheezers is indicative of an alteration of the immune system that, on the one hand, leads to the production of IgE against food antigens early and against aeroallergens later in life and, on the other hand, predisposes to the development of persistent wheezing.

Evidence that such an alteration may already be present during the first year of life in future atopic wheezers also comes from studies of circulating eosinophils and their products. Atopic wheezers have, as a group, higher prevalence of eosinophilia ($\geq 4\%$ of white blood cells), as measured randomly, than transient wheezers or infants who never wheeze.[49] Moreover, eosinophilic responses to the viral infections that cause their first episodes of wheezing are also different in future atopic wheezers when compared with transient wheezers. During these acute episodes the future atopic wheezers have been shown to have elevated eosinophil counts and increased levels of circulating eosinophil products such as eosinophil cationic protein (ECP) when compared with other wheezers.[50,51] One of the only invasive studies in which an attempt was made to separate atopic from non-atopic wheezers during the preschool years found that bronchial washes of the former had significantly elevated eosinophil counts as a proportion of total cell counts when compared with bronchial washes obtained from non-atopic wheezers.[52]

Taken together, these results suggest that atopic wheezers have an alteration of immune responsiveness that can even be detected at the time of their first episode of wheezing. This alteration (to be discussed further in Chapter 3) is the ultimate determinant of their atopic status and of their propensity to wheeze persistently into the school years.

Lung function and atopic wheezing
Measurements of lung function are quite unhelpful in distinguishing individual infants destined to be the future atopic wheezers from other wheezers (see Chapter 5). However, as a group, atopic wheezers have lower levels of lung function at the age of 6 and beyond than other groups, a finding that is quite consistent in different studies. These deficits of lung function are (often only partially) reversible with bronchodilators and with inhaled corticosteroids, but withdrawal of these treatments is associated with a return of baseline, diminished lung function in these children.[53] BHR to methacholine, histamine, cold air and other stimulants is also very often observed in these children, and severity and persistence of BHR during childhood is strongly associated with worse

prognosis, lower levels of lung function and more severe symptoms.[54] An important issue thus becomes: when does BHR start and when do changes in lung function occur in atopic wheezing? Are they the cause or the consequence of the disease?

This is a controversial issue which has yet to be resolved. One line of thought asserts that there are alterations in airway structure present in very young children before the development of asthma and that these are independent of allergic sensitization.[55] It has also been proposed, however, that the changes associated with so-called lung remodeling occur as a consequence of the disease process in asthma, and are associated with changes in lung function and increased BHR.[56] Of great interest is a recent study by Mochizuki and coworkers.[57] These researchers measured methacholine responses at a mean age of approximately 3–4 years in three groups of children: the first group was made up of children who had not had episodes of wheezing but were at high risk of developing such episodes given their personal and/or family history of asthma; the second group had already had recurrent episodes of wheezing and had a diagnosis of asthma; and the third group were considered controls. Eighteen children in the first group developed two or more episodes of wheezing during subsequent follow-up, which lasted ≥ 1 year. A second measurement of methacholine BHR was performed at the end of follow-up in all three groups. Children from the first group who developed episodes of wheezing during follow-up were all atopic and had normal BHR at the first measurement and markedly increased BHR at the end of follow-up. No changes in BHR were observed in either established asthmatics or controls: BHR remained consistently high in the former and consistently low in the latter. Although these results require confirmation, they strongly suggest that BHR develops after the incidence of wheezing in atopic wheezers. It is at present unknown if the changes in BHR observed in atopic wheezers are associated with the concomitant development of the form of airway remodeling that has been described in older atopic asthmatics. It has been difficult, however, to determine which changes in lung structure are associated with BHR and lung function deficits, and the clinical significance of markers of lung remodeling is still under dispute.

The Perth and Tucson longitudinal studies support the contention that the changes in airway function and structure observed among atopic wheezers may be the consequence and not the cause of the disease process. These studies suggest that children who are destined to become the future atopic wheezers have, as a group, levels of lung function and BHR shortly after birth that are not significantly different from those of children who will not wheeze during the first six years of life.[14,58] By 6 years of age, however, atopic wheezers have significantly diminished levels of lung function and increased BHR. A very recent longitudinal study from Manchester, UK, assessed specific airway resistance at 3 years of age in children enrolled at birth and at high risk of developing atopic wheezing.[59] It was reported that, independent of current wheezing and of parental history of asthma, children who had become sensitized to local aeroallergens by the age of 3 had significantly higher specific airway resistance than those who had not. Although values for lung function at birth were not reported, the speculation was that these changes in lung function were the consequence of an allergic inflammation occurring in these children's lungs, which would precede the development of asthma symptoms. It is of interest that in 6-year-old children, BHR to cold, dry air, has been found to predict the development of new asthma symptoms later in life, but only among children who were also skin-test positive to allergens.[60]

Taken together, these results suggest that different tests of BHR and lung function may measure different aspects of lung and airway physiology, and that some of these tests may already be altered before the incidence of atopic wheezing and others may not. They also suggest that early sensitization to allergens is associated with changes in lung function and in bronchial responsiveness that may occur either concomitantly with the development of asthma or even before asthma has developed. Of interest is the observation that allergic sensitization that occurs during the first years of life is much more strongly associated with asthma than that occurring after the first years of life[30,61] (this issue will be further discussed in Chapter 3). However, it is important to stress here that, from an epidemiological point of view, atopic wheezing appears to be a developmental disease: changes in the immune system occurring at crucial times during the establishment of mature immune responses have enduring influences on the nature of these immune responses for a lifetime. Concomitantly, these alterations in the immune system determine altered patterns of development of the lungs, the airways and the subtle mechanisms that control airway tone. Naturally, if some of the mechanisms that have been described for transient early wheezing and non-atopic wheezing are also present in individuals who are predisposed to atopic wheezing, one should expect additive or even multiplicative effects, with these subjects having the most severe and most persistent forms of the disease.

WHAT BECOMES OF THE WHEEZY INFANT AND PRESCHOOL CHILD?

At the beginning of this chapter it was noted that even when confronted with the typical wheezy infant or preschool child, the pediatrician often feels unable to answer to the parents' most pressing question, 'Does my child have asthma?'. As a result of the material presented here, is it possible to be a little more definite in answering this question or, at least, is it possible to give some statistical probability as to the outlook for the child? In truth, despite the outstanding work that has been undertaken in following cohorts of infants to determine the prevalence of wheezing in early childhood, data on the point prevalence of wheezing, the atopic status of the child and the natural history of the condition in the individual are sparse in the extreme. To complicate matters, it is evident that there is a wide variation in the incidence of wheezing between different countries and, on the whole, wheezing in infancy and early childhood appears to be about twice as common in the USA and Australia compared to Western Europe.

Looking at the data from the USA and Australia, there are certain facts that can be deduced from the cohort studies in Tucson[14] and Perth,[62] along with the International Study of Asthma and Allergies in Children (ISAAC) worldwide study of the incidence of asthma and allergy in childhood[63] that relates to the incidence of wheezing in children aged 13–14. Data from these three studies have been amalgamated to construct Figure 1.2, which attempts to show the point prevalence of wheezing in childhood at each age and the different types of wheezing that make up the total. These data apply to

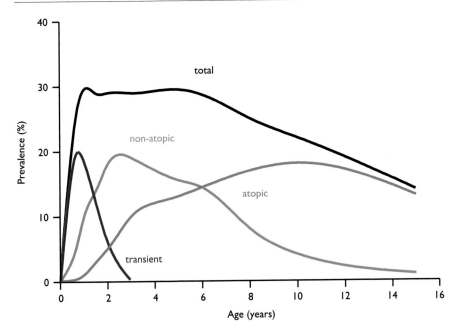

Figure 1.2

Incidence of childhood wheezing (from Martinez et al[14] and Young et al[62]).

American and Australian populations, and although the absolute numbers may be substantially less in other countries the mix of wheezing disorders is likely to be similar. In
the first year of life the total incidence of wheezing from the Perth study was 37% and in
the second year it was 33%. In the Tucson study the cumulative incidence of wheezing
in the first three years was 34%. Since some infants stop wheezing during this period,
the total point prevalence for the purposes of Figure 1.2 was taken as approximately
30% during this period. From the Tucson study it is known that some 20% of infants –
about two thirds of the total – would be transient early wheezers who are very likely to
stop wheezing in early childhood, do not carry markers of atopy and are unlikely to
become asthmatics in later childhood. By the age of 6, the Tucson study suggests a
point prevalence of wheezing of about 29%, half of whom are likely to be atopic children and half non-atopic. From then on the proportion of non-atopic wheezers steadily
decreases and the proportion of atopic wheezers steadily increases, so that by adolescence the large majority of wheezy children are typical atopic asthmatics.

So what can we really tell the parents in the light of our epidemiologic studies? We
can tell them that if their infant is about < 2 years of age then the child has a 60–70%
chance of stopping wheezing in early childhood and never developing asthma. If the
child is between the ages of about 2 and 6 then there is a better than even chance that the
wheezing is viral induced and the child is unlikely to continue to wheeze throughout
childhood or into adult life. If the child is older than about 6 years of age and still
wheezing then there is a greater chance that the problem is true atopic asthma, although

studies into adult life suggest that about at least half of these individuals will eventually lose their asthma.

As far as treatment is concerned, the atopic asthmatics clearly respond well to conventional treatment; however, there are simply no objective data as to the response to treatment of the transient early wheezy infants and the non-atopic viral-induced wheezy infants. Further studies of the response to treatment of clearly defined groups of wheezy infants and preschool children are thus required.

REFERENCES

1. Parrott RH, Kim HW, Arrobio JO et al. Epidemiology of respiratory syncytial virus infection in Washington, D.C. II. Infection and disease with respect to age, immunologic status, race and sex. Am J Epidemiol 1973; 98: 289–300.

2. Martinez FD. Sudden infant death syndrome and small airway occlusion: facts and hypothesis. Pediatrics 1991; 87: 190–8.

3. Holberg CJ, Wright AL, Martinez FD et al. Risk factors for respiratory syncytial virus-associated lower respiratory illnesses in the first year of life. Am J Epidemiol 1991; 133: 1135–51.

4. Rakes GP, Arruda E, Ingram JM et al. Rhinovirus and respiratory syncytial virus in wheezing children requiring emergency care. IgE and eosinophil analyses. Am J Resp Crit Care Med 1999; 159: 785–90.

5. Hoo AF, Dezateux C, Hanrahan JP et al. Sex-specific prediction equations for Vmax(FRC) in infancy: a multicenter collaborative study. Am J Resp Crit Care Med 2002; 165: 1084–92.

6. Kim HW, Arrobio JO, Brandt CD et al. Epidemiology of respiratory syncytial virus infection in Washington, D.C. I. Importance of the virus in different respiratory tract disease syndromes and temporal distribution of infection. Am J Epidemiol 1973; 98: 216–25.

7. Wright AL, Taussig LM, Ray CG et al. The Tucson Children's Respiratory Study. II. Lower respiratory tract illness in the first year of life. Am J Epidemiol 1989; 129: 1232–46.

8. Ray CG, Holberg CJ, Minnich LL et al. Acute lower respiratory illnesses during the first three years of life: potential roles for various etiologic agents. The Group Health Medical Associates. Pediatr Infect Dis J 1993; 12: 10–14.

9. Johnston SL, Pattemore PK, Sanderson G et al. The relationship between upper respiratory infections and hospital admissions for asthma: a time-trend analysis. Am J Resp Crit Care Med 1996; 154: 654–60.

10. Papadopoulos NG, Moustaki M, Tsolia M et al. Association of rhinovirus infection with increased disease severity in acute bronchiolitis. Am J Resp Crit Care Med 2002; 165: 1285–9.

11. Hegele RG, Ahmad HY, Becker AB et al. The association between respiratory viruses and symptoms in 2-week-old infants at high risk for asthma and allergy. J Pediatr 2001; 138: 831–7.

12. van den Hoogen BG, de Jong JC, Groen J et al. A newly discovered human pneumovirus isolated from young children with respiratory tract disease. Nat Med 2001; 7: 719–24.

13. Nissen MD, Siebert DJ, Mackay IM et al. Evidence of human metapneumovirus in Australian children. Med J Aust 2002; 176: 188.

14. Martinez FD, Wright AL, Taussig LM et al. Asthma and wheezing in the first six years of life. N Engl J Med 1995; 332: 133–8.

15. Sherriff A, Peters TJ, Henderson J, Strachan D. Risk factor associations with wheezing patterns in children followed longitudinally from birth to 3(1/2) years. Int J Epidemiol 2001; 30: 1473–84.

16. Godfrey S. The wheezy infant. In: (Meadow R, ed) *Recent Advances in Paediatrics* (Churchill Livingstone: New York, 1984) 137.

17. Boesen I. Asthmatic bronchitis in children: prognosis for 162 cases, observed 6–11 years. *Acta Paediatr* 1953; **42**: 87.

18. Rusconi F, Galassi C, Corbo GM et al. Risk factors for early, persistent, and late-onset wheezing in young children. SIDRIA Collaborative Group. *Am J Resp Crit Care Med* 1999; **160**: 1617–22.

19. Stein RT, Holberg CJ, Sherrill DL et al. The influence of parental smoking on respiratory symptoms in the first decade of life: The Tucson Children's Respiratory Study. *Am J Epidemiol* 1999; **149**: 1030–7.

20. Strachan DP, Cook DG. Health effects of passive smoking. 1. Parental smoking and lower respiratory illness in infancy and early childhood. *Thorax* 1997; **52**: 905–14.

21. Martinez FD, Morgan WJ, Wright AL et al. Diminished lung function as a predisposing factor for wheezing respiratory illness in infants. *N Engl J Med* 1988; **319**: 1112–17.

22. Dezateux C, Stocks J. Lung development and early origins of childhood respiratory illness. *Br Med Bull* 1997; **53**: 40–57.

23. Stein RT, Holberg CJ, Morgan WJ et al. Peak flow variability, methacholine responsiveness and atopy as markers for detecting different wheezing phenotypes in childhood. *Thorax* 1997; **52**: 946–52.

24. Ball TM, Castro-Rodriguez JA, Griffith KA et al. Siblings, day-care attendance, and the risk of asthma and wheezing during childhood. *N Engl J Med* 2000; **343**: 538–43.

25. Park JH, Gold DR, Spiegelman DL et al. House dust endotoxin and wheeze in the first year of life. *Am J Resp Crit Care Med* 2001; **163**: 322–8.

26. Gold DR, Burge HA, Carey V et al. Predictors of repeated wheeze in the first year of life: the relative roles of cockroach, birth weight, acute lower respiratory illness, and maternal smoking. *Am J Resp Crit Care Med* 1999; **160**: 227–36.

27. Martinez FD, Wright AL, Holberg CJ et al. Maternal age as a risk factor for wheezing lower respiratory illnesses in the first year of life. *Am J Epidemiol* 1992; **136**: 1258–68.

28. Wright AL, Holberg CJ, Martinez FD et al. Breast feeding and lower respiratory tract illness in the first year of life. *Br Med J* 1989; **299**: 946–9.

29. Burrows B, Sears MR, Flannery EM et al. Relations of bronchial responsiveness to allergy skin test reactivity, lung function, respiratory symptoms, and diagnoses in thirteen-year-old New Zealand children. *J Allergy Clin Immunol* 1995; **95**: 548–56.

30. Halonen M, Stern DA, Lohman IC et al. Two subphenotypes of childhood asthma that differ in maternal and paternal influences on asthma risk. *Am J Resp Crit Care Med* 1999; **160**: 564–70.

31. Stein RT, Sherrill D, Morgan WJ et al. Respiratory syncytial virus in early life and risk of wheeze and allergy by age 13 years. *Lancet* 1999; **353**: 541–5.

32. Veale AJ, Peat JK, Tovey ER et al. Asthma and atopy in four rural Australian aboriginal communities. *Med J Aust* 1996; **165**: 192–6.

33. Penny ME, Murad S, Madrid SS et al. Respiratory symptoms, asthma, exercise test spirometry, and atopy in schoolchildren from a Lima shanty town. *Thorax* 2001; **56**: 607–12.

34. Yemaneberhan H, Bekele Z, Venn A et al. Prevalence of wheeze and asthma and relation to atopy in urban and rural Ethiopia. *Lancet* 1997; **350**: 85–90.

35. Kattan M. Epidemiologic evidence of increased airway reactivity in children with a history of bronchiolitis. *J Pediatr* 1999; **135**: 8–13.

36. Pullen C, Hey E. Wheezing, asthma, and pulmonary dysfunction 10 years after infection with respiratory syncytial virus in infancy. *Br Med J* 1982; **5**: 1665–9.

37. Palmer LJ, Rye PJ, Gibson NA et al. Airway responsiveness in early infancy predicts asthma, lung function, and respiratory symptoms by school age. *Am J Resp Crit Care Med* 2001; **163**: 37–42.

38. Wills-Karp M. Murine models of asthma in understanding immune dysregulation in human asthma. *Immunopharmacology* 2000; **48**: 263–8.

39. Colasurdo GN, Hemming VG, Prince GA et al. Human respiratory syncytial virus produces prolonged alterations of neural control in airways of developing ferrets. *Am J Resp Crit Care Med* 1998; **157**: 1506–11.

40. Rona RJ, Gulliford MC, Chinn S. Effects of prematurity and intrauterine growth on respiratory health and lung function in childhood. *Br Med J* 1993; **306**: 817–20.

41. Steffensen FH, Sorensen HT, Gillman MW et al. Low birth weight and preterm delivery as risk factors for asthma and atopic dermatitis in young adult males. *Epidemiology* 2000; **11**: 185–8.

42. Hikino S, Nakayama H, Yamamoto J et al. Food allergy and atopic dermatitis in low birthweight infants during early childhood. *Acta Paediatr* 2001; **90**: 850–5.

43. Pelkonen AS, Hakulinen AL, Turpeinen M. Bronchial lability and responsiveness in school children born very preterm. *Am J Resp Crit Care Med* 1997; **156**: 1178–84.

44. Pelkonen AS, Hakulinen AL, Hallman M, Turpeinen M. Effect of inhaled budesonide therapy on lung function in schoolchildren born preterm. *Resp Med* 2001; **95**: 565–70.

45. Chan KN, Silverman M. Increased airway responsiveness in children of low birth weight at school age: effect of topical corticosteroids. *Arch Dis Child* 1993; **69**: 120–4.

46. Jacob SV, Coates AL, Lands LC et al. Long-term pulmonary sequelae of severe bronchopulmonary dysplasia. *J Pediatr* 1998; **133**: 193–200.

47. Burrows B, Sears MR, Flannery EM et al. Relation of the course of bronchial responsiveness from age 9 to age 15 to allergy. *Am J Resp Crit Care Med* 1995; **152**: 1302–8.

48. Illi S, von Mutius E, Lau S et al. The pattern of atopic sensitization is associated with the development of asthma in childhood. *J Allergy Clin Immunol* 2001; **108**: 709–14.

49. Karakoc F, Remes ST, Martinez FD, Wright AL. The association between persistent eosinophilia and asthma in childhood is independent of atopic status. *Clin Exp Allergy* 2002; **32**: 51–6.

50. Reijonen TM, Korppi M, Kuikka L et al. Serum eosinophil cationic protein as a predictor of wheezing after bronchiolitis. *Pediatr Pulmonol* 1997; **23**: 397–403.

51. Pifferi M, Ragazzo V, Caramella D, Baldini G. Eosinophil cationic protein in infants with respiratory syncytial virus bronchiolitis: predictive value for subsequent development of persistent wheezing. *Pediatr Pulmonol* 2001; **31**: 419–24.

52. Stevenson EC, Turner G, Heaney LG et al. Bronchoalveolar lavage findings suggest two different forms of childhood asthma. *Clin Exp Allergy* 1997; **27**: 1027–35.

53. The Childhood Asthma Management Program Research Group. Long-term effects of budesonide or nedocromil in children with asthma. *N Engl J Med* 2000; **343**: 1054–63.

54. Sears MR. Evolution of asthma through childhood. *Clin Exp Allergy* 1998; **28** (**suppl 5**): 82–9.

55. Holgate ST. Genetic and environmental interaction in allergy and asthma. *J Allergy Clin Immunol* 1999; **104**: 1139–46.

56. Martinez FD. Development of wheezing disorders and asthma in preschool children. *Pediatrics* 2002; **109** (**Suppl 2**): 362–7.

57. Mochizuki M. Bronchial hyperresponsiveness before and after the diagnosis of bronchial asthma in children. *Pediatrics* 2000; **106**: 1442–6.

58. Stick SM, Arnott J, Turner DJ et al. Bronchial responsiveness and lung function in recurrently wheezy infants. *Am Rev Resp Dis* 1991; **144**: 1012–15.

59. Lowe L, Murray CS, Custovic A et al. Specific airway resistance in 3-year-old children: a prospective cohort study. *Lancet* 2002; **359**: 1904–8.

60. Lombardi E, Morgan WJ, Wright AL et al. Cold air challenge at age 6 and

subsequent incidence of asthma. A longitudinal study. *Am J Resp Crit Care Med* 1997; **156**: 1863–9.

61. Peat JK, Salome CM, Woolcock AJ. Longitudinal changes in atopy during a 4-year period: relation to bronchial hyperresponsiveness and respiratory symptoms in a population sample of Australian schoolchildren. *J Allergy Clin Immunol* 1990; **85**: 65–74.

62. Young S, Arnott J, O'Keeffe PT et al. The association between early life lung function and wheezing during the first 2 yrs of life. *Eur Resp J* 2000; **15**: 151–7.

63. The International Study of Asthma and Allergies in Childhood (ISACC). Worldwide variation in prevalence of symptoms of asthma, allergic rhinoconjunctivitis, and atopic eczema: ISAAC. *Lancet* 1998; **351**: 1225–32.

2
Respiratory syncytial virus (RSV) infection and wheezing

INTRODUCTION

By far the most frequent cause of severe episodes of wheezing during infancy and early childhood is infection with the respiratory syncytial virus (RSV). In the USA alone approximately 100,000 hospitalizations from lower respiratory illnesses (LRI) due to RSV (RSV-LRI) occur each year[1] and approximately 500 deaths/year are attributed to these infections.[2] Although virtually all children have evidence of having had an RSV infection by the end of the second year of life,[3] only a fraction develop clinical manifestations of RSV-LRI.

CLINICAL PRESENTATIONS

Infections with RSV can have a variety of clinical presentations. As explained elsewhere, the most common presentation of symptomatic RSV infection in infants < 30–45 days of age is not direct airway involvement but central apnea.[4] This may become a life-threatening condition and may be the sole manifestation of RSV infection very early in life. What determines apnea in very young children with RSV is not understood, but premature children are particularly susceptible to this clinical manifestation. Children with apnea and confirmed RSV infection should be hospitalized and monitored closely until they remain free of apnea for at least 48 hours. Rarely do these episodes become very frequent and difficult to control, but in these rare cases, intubation and mechanical ventilation may be required.

Older infants with RSV infection usually first present with signs and symptoms of upper respiratory illness (URI), characterized by increased nasal secretions, fever, otitis and cough.[5,6] In the majority of infants, symptoms are limited to these manifestations of URI and no lower airway involvement is evident. However, studies of lung function performed during acute URI in young infants have demonstrated significant impairment in parameters of lung function usually thought to be indices of lower airway function, as assessed by the chest compression technique.[7] It is thus possible that all infants with RSV infection may have lower airway involvement, which remains clinically unapparent in most.

In approximately one third of infants infected with RSV, signs and symptoms of LRI become evident. The most common syndrome associated with LRI during RSV infection is bronchiolitis. Although there has been some dispute as to what exactly constitutes bronchiolitis, the typical infant with this syndrome is difficult to miss. After a brief period (2–5 days) of URI, these young children develop wheezing, tachypnea and retractions. Physical examination shows variable signs of hypoxemia, wheezing and rales, and evident hyperinflation. Chest films show lung hyperinflation and interstitial changes compatible with pneumonitis.

Some infants probably have more severe lower airway obstruction, with consequent atelectasis, which is manifested radiographically as patchy or frank consolidation. These infants also have more severe tachypnea, and this combination usually prompts the diagnosis of pneumonia. It is difficult, however, to determine if this is a separate syndrome altogether or is simply a more severe manifestation of the same basic condition present in bronchiolitis. In order to investigate this issue, Castro-Rodriguez et al[8] compared the risk factors for and the long-term sequelae of radiologically confirmed pneumonia with those for LRI without pneumonia occurring during the first three years of life in subjects enrolled in the Tucson Children's Respiratory Study. Proportions of children from whom RSV, parainfluenza virus or other agents were isolated for the first episode of pneumonia or for the first LRI without pneumonia was not significantly different for the two groups, with one third of all children with pneumonia having RSV infection. Both, children with pneumonia and those with LRI without pneumonia were more likely to have a diagnosis of asthma and frequent wheezing at the ages of 6 and 11 than children without a history of LRI, but the risk was much higher in those with pneumonia than in those with LRI without pneumonia; children with pneumonia and those with LRI without pneumonia had diminished levels of lung function shortly after birth and before any LRI developed. Both also had lower levels of indices derived from the second half of the forced expiratory flow–volume curve at the ages of 6 and 11 years when compared with children without a history of LRI, but children with a history of pneumonia had the largest deficits. At the age of 11, both for pneumonia and LRI without pneumonia, deficits in lung function were significantly reversed after administration of a bronchodilator. The authors concluded that the deficits in lung function observed in these two conditions were, to a significant extent, due to alterations in the regulation of airway tone. These findings suggest that there is a continuum of severity of RSV-LRI in early life, and that pneumonia and bronchiolitis are part of that continuum.

It is important to stress that young children with RSV infection may also present with croup-like symptoms.[9] Although this presentation is rarer than the three described above, it is not uncommon in older (2–3-year-old) children. This clinical presentation suggests that in most cases of RSV, the entire respiratory epithelium is involved and may determine the development of symptoms that are specific to different airway levels. The clinician needs to consider the possibility, therefore, that obstruction of the upper, central and lower airways may increase the severity of RSV illness and may require treatment that is specific for each type of obstruction.

DIAGNOSIS

Diagnosis of RSV infection is usually straightforward and is based on clinical presentation and seasonality. In such children, laboratory examinations (apart from viral studies) are usually unnecessary and should be avoided. In children with severe disease and in whom hospitalization is being considered, a chest radiograph may be useful to rule out pneumonia or other complications.

In individuals who are suspected of having RSV illness, etiologic studies to ascertain the presence of such illness may be indicated but are by no means mandatory, given the lack of any widely accepted specific treatment for RSV. In young children at high risk, and even among those with mild disease, confirmation that an acute respiratory illness is due to RSV may be necessary so as to allow the clinician to make decisions regarding the use of certain medications (see below) or the need for more careful monitoring. Nasal secretions are most frequently used for a definitive diagnosis in children with a presumptive diagnosis of RSV infection, because RSV is almost invariably present in nasal mucosa during such infections, regardless of the clinical presentation. Secretions can be obtained either by nasopharyngeal washings or aspiration. Two rapid identification techniques are commercially available: direct and indirect fluorescent antibodies. In the direct technique, antibodies bind to RSV and appear as luminescence on the surface of epithelial cells obtained from secretions and fixed on slide preparations. In the indirect technique, enzyme immunoassays detect RSV by using enzyme-conjugated, anti-RSV antibodies. The direct technique has both sensitivity and specificity > 90%, whereas these values are slightly lower for the different enzyme immunoassays available. Tests based on reverse-transcriptase-polymerase chain reaction (PCR) have also become available,[10] and they allow distinction of the two RSV subtypes, A and B.

EPIDEMIOLOGY

RSV infection is usually seasonal, with outbreaks that often begin in late fall and extend into early spring, although isolation of RSV is not unheard of during the summer months. RSV is apparently only a human pathogen and transmission occurs either directly through inhalation of airborne droplets or by inoculation through the hands of adults caring for young children. RSV can survive for almost half an hour on unwashed hands and up to six hours on household surfaces.[11] Inoculation almost invariably occurs through the nose and eyes.[12] The incubation period is approximately five days.

The factors that determine why some children develop clinical signs of lower airway obstruction and wheezing during RSV infection have been discussed elsewhere in this book. Several factors are known to increase the likelihood of severe RSV-LRI requiring hospitalization (Box 2.1). From the point of view of public health, the most influential among these factors is prematurity, which accounts for 24% of all hospitalizations due to RSV.[13] Congenital heart disease (17%) and chronic lung disease (13%) account for the bulk of the remaining ascertainable risk factors for severe RSV-LRI. Less important from the point of view of morbidity, but not certainly from that of mortality, are underlying immunosuppressive conditions such as acquired immunodeficiency syndrome, (AIDS)[14] and congenital immunodeficiency, and children who have received chemotherapy and those who have undergone organ transplantation.[15,16] Children who are not breastfed, those who were exposed to tobacco-smoke products *in utero* or are currently exposed to environmental tobacco smoke or to non-tobacco indoor smoke

---

Box 2.1 Risk factors for severe lower respiratory illness due to the respiratory syncytial virus (RSV-LRI)

Prematurity
Age < 2 months
Congenital heart disease
Respiratory muscle impairment (due to muscular dystrophy or other genetic or metabolic conditions)
Acquired immunodeficiency syndrome (AIDS)
Congenital immunodeficiencies
Organ transplantation
Treatment with chemotherapy
Chronic lung disease of prematurity (and other chronic lung diseases)
Infants with multiple congenital anomalies

---

pollution, those who live in crowded quarters or who have several older siblings are all at increased risk for RSV-LRI.[17–20]

Of particular significance is the increased risk of severe RSV-LRI observed among Native American populations in the USA, with hospitalization rates nearly twice as high as those observed among other children in the same country.[21] It is at present not known if this higher risk of severe RSV-LRI is due to an increased prevalence of some of the risk factors described above or if Native American populations show increased prevalence of genetic factors associated with RSV-LRI.

Respiratory infections due to RSV are one of the main causes of morbidity and mortality of young children in poor countries of the world.[22] Although the factors that determine this increased burden have not been specifically studied, it is reasonable to surmise that crowding, malnutrition and poor hygienic conditions are important contributors. Since massive vaccination strategies have been successful in decreasing other infectious diseases in poor countries, the development of an effective RSV immunization would be a major breakthrough for public health worldwide. Unfortunately, efforts to develop such immunization have not yet been successful, but use of modern genomic technologies is offering promising new avenues in this field.[23]

Children with confirmed RSV-LRI are at significant increased risk of subsequent development of recurrent episodes of wheezing.[24,25] The potential role of RSV-LRI in the development of atopic and non-atopic wheezing later in life is discussed in detail elsewhere in this book (Chapter 1).

GENETICS

There is very little information regarding the potential role of genetic factors in determining susceptibility to RSV-LRI. No studies in the literature have compared the risk of RSV-LRI in siblings of children who had RSV-LRI with that in siblings of children who did not have RSV-LRI. Surprisingly, no published studies have compared concordance for RSV-LRI in monozygotic and dizygotic twins, which is the method of choice to determine the role of genetic factors in disease susceptibility in humans. Comparisons of different strains of inbred mice suggest that genetic factors play a role in determining RSV titers after standard experimental inoculation,[26] but the relevance of these experiments for humans remains elusive, given the fact that humans are the only known natural reservoir for RSV.

Reports of the association between incidence of RSV-LRI and polymorphisms in potential candidate genes for the illness are scanty. In one such study, Hull et al[27] screened for genetic variants in the promoter region of the gene for interleukin (IL)-8. A group of children who had been admitted for RSV bronchiolitis was subsequently genotyped for one such polymorphism. Promoter regions of all genes usually regulate the rate of transcription of the gene, and thus the amount of protein that is synthesized by the cell. The authors chose IL-8 because it is a potent attractant for neutrophils, which appear to be the predominant cell in bronchoalveolar lavage (BAL) of children with RSV bronchiolitis.[28,29] In addition, clinical studies have identified high levels of IL-8 in plasma and nasal secretions of infants with RSV bronchiolitis.[30] The main finding of the study was that the A allele for a polymorphism located 251 bases upstream from the transcription start site of the gene was transmitted by parents to their children with RSV-LRI significantly more frequently than was expected by chance. Although the results of this study require confirmation, it appears that variants for IL-8 may play a significant role in the genetic susceptibility to severe RSV-LRI.

TREATMENT

There is no specific treatment for RSV-LRI that is universally accepted and used by all major academic and clinical centers worldwide. This absence of proven effective therapy for a severe respiratory illness that affects so many young children is quite frustrating for the clinician who cares for these children and for their parents. For this reason, many clinicians attempt different empirical treatments known to be effective in other illnesses that are clinically similar to or epidemiologically related to RSV (e.g. asthma of the older child).

Oxygen and supportive care

All children hospitalized with RSV bronchiolitis have some degree of chest hyperinflation and, as a consequence, are likely to have significant maldistribution of ventilation and ventilation–perfusion mismatch. Thus, all admitted infants with confirmed RSV should receive supplemental oxygen by way of a hood or, if symptoms and hypoxemia are particularly severe, by use of a face mask or nasal cannula. This is the single most effective and least costly treatment for severe RSV-LRI.

Children with severe RSV-LRI should be kept in quiet environments. Chest physiotherapy is usually not required and may be counterproductive in very young children with severe airway obstruction. Although hydration is important, most infants with RSV-LRI can be fed orally and do not require more than maintenance fluids, if that. Unnecessary procedures and stimulation should be avoided, although close attention should be paid to respiratory effort and oxygen saturation status. Children with confirmed RSV should preferentially be housed with no other uninfected young child, given the high likelihood of the latter becoming infected by direct contact or by transmission through hospital personnel.

Bronchodilators

Beta-2-adrenergic agonists (β_2-agonists) are routinely used for the treatment of RSV-LRI in many centers, but the effectiveness of these drugs for the treatment of airway obstruction in this age group has not been established.[31] Both clinical outcomes[32–34] and results of pulmonary function tests[35–37] have been used to determine the potential usefulness of β_2-agonists. Results have been inconclusive, with some studies showing some relief,[32,38] others no changes in mean clinical scores[34] and others showing functional deterioration in some children.[35,36] These findings and empirical clinical observations suggest that there is indeed a group of children who may improve with the use of inhaled bronchodilators, but that infants with acute RSV-LRI do not show the same kind of responses to β_2-agonists observed in older children with asthma. Therefore, a clinical trial of β_2-agonists by inhalation appears justified in all infants with RSV, particularly considering the fact that potential adverse reactions to β_2-agonists are usually not severe and are short lasting. Nevertheless, persisting in the use of β_2-agonists in high doses in infants with RSV-LRI who have not responded to this therapy is counterproductive and cannot be justified.

Inhaled epinephrine

Clinical trials using inhaled racemic epinephrine[34,39,40] have suggested that some children may respond to this therapy with significant, albeit short-lasting, improvements in lung function tests and in clinical scores. The implication of these studies is that the mechanism of action of epinephrine is different from that of β_2-agonists, and perhaps related not to bronchodilation but to a decrease in airway edema, especially in the upper airway. It is important to recall here that some infants with RSV have signs and symptoms of laryngeal obstruction,[9] and it is possible that some involvement of the laryngeal mucosa may be present in many infants with acute RSV infection. What role this may play in the improvement associated with the use of epinephrine in these children is unknown. Based on these considerations, it is also reasonable to attempt a trial therapy with inhaled epinephrine in infants with acute airway obstruction.

Corticosteroids

Many studies, both randomized and non-randomized, have been published in which both oral and inhaled corticosteroids were used during the acute phase of RSV-LRI.[41,42] Taken as a whole, the results of these studies do not support the systematic use of corticosteroids in infants with RSV infection. Because these studies included infants with RSV without regard for potential heterogeneity in the disease mechanisms associated with the illness, it is still possible that certain subgroups of children with RSV-LRI may respond to the use of corticosteroids. However, no reliable markers that could be used to identify such children are currently available.

Ribavirin

During the mid-1980s there was considerable interest in the potential use of antiviral agents for the treatment of acute RSV. Ribavirin is the only such agent currently approved for use during RSV infections. Although initial studies seemed to suggest a significant effect of ribavirin on the short-term outcome of RSV infection,[43] the impression of many experienced clinicians is that these effects are, at best, modest and require the use of this drug quite early on during the course of the illness. Moreover, doubts have also emerged regarding the methodologies used in some of the original studies used to demonstrate the effectiveness of ribavirin in RSV illness. For these reasons, the American Academy of Pediatrics revised its original recommendations and restricted the use of ribavirin to infants at very high risk for serious RSV disease.[44]

PREVENTION

Based on the fact that there is no universally effective treatment for acute RSV infection in infants, the potential role of preventive approaches to RSV illness have gained significant ground among the scientific community and in the pharmaceutical industry. Vaccine development has encountered major obstacles, and initial attempts with formalin-inactivated virus were associated with disastrous increases in morbidity and mortality associated with RSV illness.[45] For these reasons, research and drug development efforts have focused on passive immunization by use of specific antibodies against RSV and two approaches are available.

RSV intravenous immunoglobulins (Respigam)

These products are prepared from donors selected for high titers of anti-RSV antibodies.[46] In the USA, this product is licensed for use in children < 24 months of age with a history of bronchopulmonary dysplasia or preterm birth (< 36 weeks gestation). Although this treatment has proven to be effective in the prevention of severe RSV,[47] intravenous administration needs to occur every month, for 5 months, during the season for acute RSV. Due the fact that it may contain other antibodies apart from those against RSV, intravenous immunoglobulin can also interfere with common vaccinations such as the measles, mumps and rubella (MMR) vaccine.

Monoclonal antibodies against RSV (palivizumab, Synagis)

Palivizumab is a humanized mouse monoclonal antibody against one of the constitutive proteins of RSV, the F protein. It also needs to be given monthly, but has the advantage that it is administered subcutaneously and does not interfere with the vaccination process.

Since studies of the efficacy of these two products have not shown a particular advantage of one over the other, palivizumab is more widely used given its ease of administration and lack of interference with immunizations. Currently, palivizumab is used only for prevention purposes in high risk infants[48] and not for treatment of acute RSV illness.

REFERENCES

1. Shay DK, Holman RC, Newman RD et al. Bronchiolitis-associated hospitalizations among US children, 1980–1996. *J Am Med Assoc* 1999; **282**: 1440–6.

2. Shay DK, Holman RC, Roosevelt GE et al. Bronchiolitis-associated mortality and estimates of respiratory syncytial virus-associated deaths among US children, 1979–1997. *J Inf Dis* 2001; **183**: 16–22.

3. Glezen WP, Taber LH, Frank AL, Kasel JA. Risk of primary infection and reinfection with respiratory syncytial virus. *Am J Dis Child* 1986; **140**: 543–6.

4. Kneyber MC, Brandenburg AH, de Groot R et al. Risk factors for respiratory syncytial virus associated apnoea. *Eur J Pediatr* 1998; **157**: 331–5.

5. Heikkinen T, Thint M, Chonmaitree T. Prevalence of various respiratory viruses in the middle ear during acute otitis media. *N Engl J Med* 1999; **340**: 260–4 (comment).

6. Henderson FW, Collier AM, Clyde Jr WA, Denny FW. Respiratory-syncytial-virus infections, reinfections and immunity. A prospective, longitudinal study in young children. *N Engl J Med* 1979; **300**: 530–4.

7. Martinez FD, Taussig LM, Morgan WJ. Infants with upper respiratory illnesses have significant reductions in maximal expiratory flow. *Pediatr Pulmonol* 1990; **9**: 91–5.

8. Castro-Rodriguez JA, Holberg CJ, Wright AL et al. Association of radiologically ascertained pneumonia before age 3 yr with asthma-like symptoms and pulmonary function during childhood: a prospective study. *Am J Resp Crit Care Med* 1999; **159**: 1891–7.

9. Castro-Rodriguez JA, Holberg CJ, Morgan WJ et al. Relation of two different subtypes of croup before age three to wheezing, atopy, and pulmonary function during childhood: a prospective study. *Pediatrics* 2001; **107**: 512–18.

10. Falsey AR, Formica MA, Walsh EE. Diagnosis of respiratory syncytial virus infection: comparison of reverse transcription-PCR to viral culture and serology in adults with respiratory illness. *J Clin Microbiol* 2002; **40**: 817–20.

11. Hall CB, Douglas Jr RG, Geiman JM. Possible transmission by fomites of respiratory syncytial virus. *J Inf Dis* 1980; **141**: 98–102.

12. Hall CB, Douglas Jr RG, Schnabel KC, Geiman JM. Infectivity of respiratory syncytial virus by various routes of inoculation. *Inf Immun* 1981; **33**: 779–83.

13. Navas L, Wang E, de Carvalho V, Robinson J. Improved outcome of respiratory syncytial virus infection in a high-risk hospitalized population of Canadian children. Pediatric Investigators Collaborative Network on Infections in Canada. *J Pediatr* 1992; **121**: 348–54.

14. Madhi SA, Venter M, Madhi A et al. Differing manifestations of respiratory syncytial virus-associated severe lower respiratory tract infections in human immunodeficiency virus type 1-infected and uninfected children. *Pediatr Inf Dis J* 2001; **20**: 164–70.

15. McCarthy AJ, Kingman HM, Kelly C et al. The outcome of 26 patients with respiratory syncytial virus infection following allogeneic stem cell transplantation. *Bone Marrow Transplant* 1999; **24**: 1315–22.

16. Wendt CH, Hertz MI. Respiratory syncytial virus and parainfluenza virus infections in the immunocompromised host. *Semin Resp Inf* 1995; **10**: 224–31.

17. Holberg CJ, Wright AL, Martinez FD et al. Risk factors for respiratory syncytial virus-associated lower respiratory illnesses in

the first year of life. *Am J Epidemiol* 1991; **133**: 1135–51.

18. Wright AL, Taussig LM, Ray CG et al. The Tucson Children's Respiratory Study. II. Lower respiratory tract illness in the first year of life. *Am J Epidemiol* 1989; **129**: 1232–46.

19. Wright AL, Holberg CJ, Martinez FD et al. Breast feeding and lower respiratory tract illness in the first year of life. *Br Med J* 1989; **299**: 946–9.

20. Law BJ, Carbonell-Estrany X, Simoes EA. An update on respiratory syncytial virus epidemiology: a developed country perspective. *Res Med* 2002; **96 (suppl B)**: S1–S7.

21. Bockova J, O'Brien KL, Oski J et al. Respiratory syncytial virus infection in Navajo and White Mountain Apache children. *Pediatrics* 2002; **110**: 20.

22. Weber MW, Mulholland EK, Greenwood BM. Respiratory syncytial virus infection in tropical and developing countries. *Trop Med Int Health* 1998; **3**: 268–80.

23. Collins PL, Murphy BR. Respiratory syncytial virus: reverse genetics and vaccine strategies. *Virology* 2002; **296**: 204–11.

24. Stein RT, Sherrill D, Morgan WJ et al. Respiratory syncytial virus in early life and risk of wheeze and allergy by age 13 years. *Lancet* 1999; **353**: 541–5.

25. Sigurs N, Bjarnason R, Sigurbergsson F, Kjellman B. Respiratory syncytial virus bronchiolitis in infancy is an important risk factor for asthma and allergy at age 7. *Am J Resp Crit Care Med* 2000; **161**: 1501–7.

26. Stark JM, McDowell SA, Koenigsknecht V et al. Genetic susceptibility to respiratory syncytial virus infection in inbred mice. *J Med Virol* 2002; **67**: 92–100.

27. Hull J, Thomson A, Kwiatkowski D. Association of respiratory syncytial virus bronchiolitis with the interleukin 8 gene region in UK families. *Thorax* 2000; **55**: 1023–7.

28. Smith PK, Wang SZ, Dowling KD, Forsyth KD. Leucocyte populations in respiratory syncytial virus-induced bronchiolitis. *J Paediatr Child Health* 2001; **37**: 146–51.

29. Jones A, Qui JM, Bataki E et al. Neutrophil survival is prolonged in the airways of healthy infants and infants with RSV bronchiolitis. *Eur Respir J* 2002; **20**: 651–7.

30. Sheeran P, Jafri H, Carubelli C et al. Elevated cytokine concentrations in the nasopharyngeal and tracheal secretions of children with respiratory syncytial virus disease. *Pediatr Inf Dis J* 1999; **18**: 115–22.

31. Kornecki A, Shemie SD. Bronchodilators and RSV-induced respiratory failure: agonizing about beta2 agonists. *Pediatr Pulmonol* 1998; **26**: 4–5 (comment).

32. Klassen TP, Rowe PC, Sutcliffe T et al. Randomized trial of salbutamol in acute bronchiolitis. *J Pediatr* 1991; **118**: 807–11. (Erratum appears in *J Pediatr* 1991; **119**: 1010).

33. Ho L, Collis G, Landau LI, Le Souef PN. Effect of salbutamol on oxygen saturation in bronchiolitis. *Arch Dis Child* 1991; **66**: 1061–4.

34. Patel H, Platt R, Pekeles G, Ducharme F. A randomized, controlled trial of the effectiveness of nebulized therapy with epinephrine compared with albuterol and saline in infants hospitalized for acute viral bronchiolitis. *J Pediatr* 2002; **141**: 818–24.

35. Prendiville A, Green S, Silverman M. Paradoxical response to nebulised salbutamol in wheezy infants, assessed by partial expiratory flow–volume curves. *Thorax* 1987; **42**: 86–91.

36. Hughes DM, Lesouef PN, Landau LI. Effect of salbutamol on respiratory mechanics in bronchiolitis. *Pediatr Res* 1987; **22**: 83–6.

37. Rutter N, Milner AD, Hiller EJ. Effect of bronchodilators on respiratory resistance in infants and young children with bronchiolitis and wheezy bronchitis. *Arch Dis Child* 1975; **50**: 719–22.

38. Schuh S, Canny G, Reisman JJ et al. Nebulized albuterol in acute bronchiolitis. *J Pediatr* 1990; **117**: 633–7.

39. Bertrand P, Aranibar H, Castro E, Sanchez I. Efficacy of nebulized epinephrine versus salbutamol in hospitalized

infants with bronchiolitis. *Pediatr Pulmonol* 2001; **31**: 284–8.

40.   Sanchez I, De Koster J, Powell RE et al. Effect of racemic epinephrine and salbutamol on clinical score and pulmonary mechanics in infants with bronchiolitis. *J Pediatr* 1993; **122**: 145–51 (comment).

41.   van Woensel J, Kimpen J. Therapy for respiratory tract infections caused by respiratory syncytial virus. *Eur J Pediatr* 2000; **159**: 391–8.

42.   Cade A, Brownlee KG, Conway SP et al. Randomised placebo controlled trial of nebulised corticosteroids in acute respiratory syncytial viral bronchiolitis. *Arch Dis Child* 2000; **82**: 126–30.

43.   Hall CB, McBride JT, Walsh EE et al. Aerosolized ribavirin treatment of infants with respiratory syncytial viral infection. A randomized double-blind study. *N Engl J Med* 1983; **308**: 1443–7.

44.   Anonymous. Reassessment of the indications for ribavirin therapy in respiratory syncytial virus infections. American Academy of Pediatrics Committee on Infectious Diseases. *Pediatrics* 1996; **97**: 137–40.

45.   Kim HW, Canchola JG, Brandt CD et al. Respiratory syncytial virus disease in infants despite prior administration of antigenic inactivated vaccine. *Am J Epidemiol* 1969; **89**: 422–34.

46.   Staat MA. Respiratory syncytial virus infections in children. *Semin Resp Inf* 2002; **17**: 15–20.

47.   Anonymous. Reduction of respiratory syncytial virus hospitalization among premature infants and infants with bronchopulmonary dysplasia using respiratory syncytial virus immune globulin prophylaxis. The PREVENT Study Group. *Pediatrics* 1997; **99**: 93–9 (comment).

48.   Anonymous. Palivizumab, a humanized respiratory syncytial virus monoclonal antibody, reduces hospitalization from respiratory syncytial virus infection in high-risk infants. The IMpact–RSV Study Group. *Pediatrics* 1998; **102**: 531–7.

3
Immunology of wheezing disorders in infants and preschool children

IMMUNOLOGY OF WHEEZING NOT RELATED TO ATOPY

As discussed in other chapters of this book, wheezing not related to atopy is the most frequent condition associated with recurrent airway obstruction during infancy and early childhood. However, in spite of its public health impact, little was known until recently about the immune factors associated with this form of wheezing. With the advent of flexible fiberoptic bronchoscopy and modern technologies for the study of immune responses by white blood cells, new insights about the possible immunologic factors involved in wheezing not related to atopy have emerged. In epidemiologic studies, the two presentations of wheezing not related to atopy in early life, transient early wheezing and non-atopic wheezing, can be distinguished from the point of view of their risk factors and prognosis (see Chapter 1), and it is possible and likely that different immune mechanisms may be involved in their pathogenesis. Unfortunately, most available studies of wheezing among preschoolers were either retrospective or cross-sectional in design, and this precluded precise distinctions between transient early wheezing and non-atopic wheezing. In this section, published information regarding the potential immune mechanisms involved in either or both these two forms, as opposed to those presumably involved in atopic wheezing, will be reviewed. The immune mechanisms that determine immune responses to respiratory syncytial virus (RSV) during acute lower respiratory illness (LRI) are discussed separately (see Chapter 2).

Studies of bronchial samples

There is quite consistent evidence suggesting that the type of inflammation present in the lungs of young children with non-atopic forms of recurrent wheezing is different from that observed in older children with asthma. Stevenson et al[1] performed non-bronchoscopic bronchoalveolar lavage (BAL) in preschool children and found that children with non-atopic wheezing did not show the increases in proportions of mast cells and eosinophils that were present in atopic wheezers from the same age group. Since the study was done away from acute wheezing, the results indicated that ongoing inflammation was present in both forms of wheezing, but with different underlying mechanisms. The authors did not classify non-atopic wheezers by age, and thus it was not possible to know if non-atopic wheezers aged < 3 years of age (e.g. with predominance of transient wheezers) had a different cell profile from that observed in children

≥ 3 years of age. Marguet et al[2] studied 26 children < 4 years of age with infantile wheezing and 14 children > 4 years of age with asthma. They found that BAL fluid of infantile wheezers had proportionally more neutrophils whereas asthmatics had proportionally more eosinophils than control children without a history of wheezing. Le Bourgeois et al[3] recently reported results of BAL in children < 3 years of age with recurrent, severe episodes of wheezing unresponsive to inhaled corticosteroids. They found that, when compared with controls, these children had significantly higher proportions of neutrophils but not of eosinophils in BAL fluid. The larger number of neutrophils in children with wheezing was not correlated with bacterial or viral infection, or with age, sex or atopic status. Krawiec et al[4] also performed bronchoscopic BAL in children with persistent wheezing < 5 years of age and away from acute disease. When compared with controls of similar age but with no history of respiratory disease, persistent wheezers showed signs of chronic airway inflammation. All cell-type counts were increased in the latter, but the concentrations (as a percentage of total cells) were not significantly higher for any cell type in persistent wheezers compared with controls. Taken together, these studies suggest that non-atopic wheezers do have a chronic form of airway inflammation that is different from that of atopic wheezers in the same age group, and that this inflammation is usually characterized by the presence of increased numbers and proportions of neutrophils but not eosinophils.

What determines this chronic inflammation in non-atopic wheezers is not well understood. Krawiec et al[4] found that the concentrations of 15-hydroxyeicosatetraenoic acid (HETE), prostaglandin E2, and leukotrienes B4 and E4 were increased in BAL of persistent wheezers when compared with controls. Similarly, Azevedo et al[5,6] observed that spontaneous release of tumor necrosis factor-alpha (TNF-α), thromboxane A2 and leukotriene B4 was much higher in alveolar macrophages obtained from children < 3 years of age with recurrent wheezing than in controls. These same authors also reported that eosinophilic cationic protein (ECP) was increased in the BAL of young children with recurrent wheezing, but interestingly these levels did not correlate with the proportion of eosinophils in BAL but with that of neutrophils.[6] Since both neutrophils and eosinophils are able to secrete ECP, the authors speculated that the former could be the source of ECP in wheezing young children. These studies thus indicated that, even when symptom free, many young children with recurrent wheezing episodes (presumably with a majority of transient wheezers and non-atopic wheezers among them) have alveolar macrophages that seem to be in a state of persistent activation, and release increased amounts of pro-inflammatory mediators. They also show that products of other cells such as neutrophils may play a role in the pathogenesis of non-atopic wheezing.

Interferon gamma (INF-γ) and interleukin (IL) 4 responses by peripheral blood mononuclear cells (PBMC)

The potential role of alterations in immune regulation in non-atopic wheezers that may not be limited to the lungs and airways, and involve the immune system as a whole, has only recently been explored. Koning et al[7] studied preschool children with recurrent episodes of wheezing who were either atopic or non-atopic as assessed by the presence of specific immunoglobulin E (IgE) against food or aeroallergens in their serum. They found that non-atopic wheezers had significantly lower IFN-γ responses by non-specifically stimulated, purified T-cells obtained from peripheral blood as compared with healthy subjects of the same age. This was different from what was observed among children with atopic wheezing who had normal IFN-γ responses by isolated T-cells. IL-4 production by stimulated T-cells, on the other hand, was elevated in atopic wheezers as compared with controls. Leech et al[8] also studied non-specifically stimulated T-cells in atopic and non-atopic wheezy children, but from an older age group (between the ages of 5 and 15). They again reported that both CD4-positive T-cells (helper T-cells) and CD8-positive (cytotoxic T-cells) from non-atopic wheezers produced significantly less IFN-γ than those from normal controls, whereas the same cells obtained from atopic wheezers produced levels of IFN-γ that were not significantly different from those of controls. In these older children, however, IL-4 production was not increased in either group of wheezers as compared with controls. These two studies point in the same direction: non-atopic wheezers have diminished IFN-γ production regardless of age. However, they do not allow us to determine if these abnormalities existed before the development of recurrent, non-atopic wheezing or if they are the consequence of the disease process associated with chronic airway inflammation in these subjects. Unfortunately, very scanty data are available in which IFN-γ responses were assessed before the development of any LRI in children. A preliminary report from the Tucson Infant Immune Study suggests that IFN-γ responses by PBMC at 3 months of age are indeed inversely related to the subsequent development of recurrent wheezing during the first year of life (unpublished observations). If these results are confirmed, it may mean that one potential derangement present in non-atopic wheezing may be a persistent, innate alteration in the capacity of the immune system to respond to the main agent causing this form of wheezing, namely viral infection. How these findings may relate to the alteration observed in lung cells of non-atopic wheezers is unknown. Reduced IFN-γ production by T-cells may alter the regulation of macrophage responses to viral infection, or may enhance neutrophilic responses and chronic airway inflammation by increasing the likelihood that the viruses may become more invasive and less likely to be cleared from the lung.

Potential role of other cytokines

Although studies of lung cells and fluids and of PBMC have contributed important new information to our understanding of non-atopic wheeze, it is quite likely that more than one immune mechanism may contribute to the development of this condition. As explained earlier, and given the fact that we do not really know the chain of events involved in the development of non-atopic wheezing, it is not possible to know if the alterations in IFN-γ responsiveness described earlier are the consequence of the disease process or of other immune derangements. Another factor that needs to be considered is the potential for immune mediators to have effects not only on other immune cells but on non-immune cells as well. A cogent example is the recent observations by Bont et al.[9] These authors studied responses by non-specifically stimulated PBMC in children infected and hospitalized with RSV. They then compared these responses in children who did or did not have recurrent episodes of wheezing during the subsequent year.

They reported that subsequent wheezing was not related to IL-12 or IFN-γ responses at the time of the acute illness or during convalescence. However, IL-10 responses were significantly higher during the convalescent phase of the RSV infection in children who subsequently wheezed than in those who did not, and the number of subsequent wheezing episodes strongly correlated with the magnitude of the IL-10 responses. The mechanism by which IL-10 responses could predispose to recurrent wheezing subsequent to RSV infection is not known. IL-10 is known to be a potent downregulator of helper T-cells and cytotoxic T-cell responses, and this may explain, at least partially, why, for example, IFN-γ responses are diminished in non-atopic wheezers. This mechanism would suggest, therefore, that the altered IFN-γ responses are not primary but secondary to alterations of other cytokines. Perhaps different mechanisms are involved in different children, with some having primary IFN-γ abnormalities and others primary IL-10 abnormalities.

But IL-10 does not only have effects on immune cells. In animal models of RSV infection, exposure to high levels of IL-10 seems to be associated with development of an alteration in the regulation of airway tone.[10] This has been explained by a potential direct effect of IL-10 on airway smooth muscle, because exogenous IL-10 administration to naive airway smooth muscle cells elicited augmented contractility to acetylcholine and impaired relaxation to isoproterenol.[11] Therefore, in certain children, increased IL-10 responses during acute viral infections may increase airway hyperresponsiveness by acting directly on the regulation of airway smooth muscle tone, independent of any other immune mechanism, allergic or non-allergic.

Different immune mechanisms may lead to non-atopic wheezing

A conclusion that can be derived from this discussion is that different mechanisms may lead to recurrent episodes of wheezing not related to atopy during the preschool years. In certain children, an excessive immune response to viral infections, probably mediated by persistent activation of macrophages, may lead to chronic airway inflammation, which in the case of non-atopic wheezing appears to be of a neutrophilic nature. During this early life period, factors that enhance acute responses to viruses, such as certain allergens (house dust mites and cockroaches) or bacterial products (such as endotoxin), may increase the incidence of wheezing non-specifically (i.e. not through production of specific IgE) by further stimulating the release of inflammatory mediators in the lung during viral infections.[12] It is tempting to speculate that this mechanism preferentially affects transient wheezers but, unfortunately, there is no direct demonstration that this is the case. However, Litonjua et al[12] recently showed that endotoxin exposure is associated with increased risk of wheezing at 14 months of age but not at 22 and 34 months of age. At 46 months of age, children exposed to low levels of endotoxin were slightly more likely to wheeze than those exposed to high levels of endotoxin. One potential explanation for these changes could be that endotoxin exposure increases the likelihood of transient wheezing but not other forms of wheezing, although this hypothesis was not specifically tested in this study.

Children who produce an excess of IL-10 during RSV infections may also be at increased risk of subsequent recurrent wheezing by a mechanism that may directly affect airway smooth muscle contractility. However, as will be discussed more extensively later in this chapter, the main mechanism associated with non-atopic wheezing appears to be the presence of a congenital or acquired decreased IFN-γ responsiveness to viruses, which may be a common initial pathway for both atopic and non-atopic forms of wheezing in early life.

IMMUNOLOGY OF ATOPIC WHEEZING

Although atopic wheezing is not the most common condition associated with recurrent wheezing during infancy and early childhood, there is no doubt that it is the one associated with the worst long-term prognosis (see Chapter 1). Most children in whom recurrent wheezing episodes during the toddler years are associated with an allergic diathesis continue to wheeze during the school years, and there is marked tracking of symptoms during childhood.[13] Moreover, atopic wheezing is less likely to remit during the adolescent years and shows high levels of persistence of symptoms into adulthood.[14] Although most children who wheeze during the first years of life will not go on to develop the chronic forms of the disease, it is of particular interest that in the most severe cases of chronic asthma, symptoms usually begin during the first years of life.[15] For these reasons, understanding the immunological factors that determine the beginnings of atopic wheezing in infancy and its subsequent progression is important both for clinicians and researchers interested in this condition.

The purpose of this section is not to review all immunological aspects of atopic wheezing, which would go beyond the scope and extension of this book. The main objective is to study the immunology of the inception of this condition in early life. The basic premise in this chapter is that the chronic changes that are seen in atopic wheezing [allergic sensitization, bronchial hyperresponsiveness (BHR), diminished lung function, recurrent episodes of airway obstruction, persistence into adolescence and adult life] are determined by a complex combination of both genetic and environmental factors that produce alterations in the development of the immune system, the lungs and airways.

Is atopic wheezing 'caused' by allergens?

By definition, atopic wheezing is a condition in which recurrent episodes of airway obstruction are associated with evidence of sensitization against local aeroallergens. This is what differentiates it from non-atopic wheezing, the implication being that these two forms of wheezing have different pathogenetic mechanisms. For years, the basic understanding has been that wheezing and atopy are causally related, and the concept of the atopic march emerged (Figure 3.1). First, the susceptible individual is sensitized against allergens (becomes atopic). This thus supposes that a genetic susceptibility to allergies precedes and is necessary for the inception of asthma. Once this process has occurred, the individual has two possibilities: either he/she is predisposed to having BHR or some alteration in airway tone or airway structure, and in that case he/she develops wheezing; or the individual is not predisposed to BHR, in

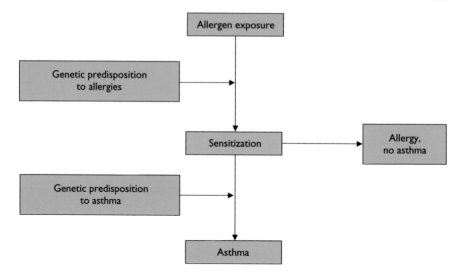

Figure 3.1

Traditional view of the association between the development of atopy and the development of asthma (atopic march).

which case he/she will only develop upper airway symptoms such as allergic rhinitis or sinusitis.

There is certainly good empirical evidence to support the contention that this could be the mechanism in many cases of asthma in older children and adults. Some individuals with asthma are monosensitized, i.e. they have evidence of circulating specific IgE against one aeroallergen and most of their symptoms are very specifically related to exposure to that aeroallergen. A large body of literature has also developed on animal models of asthma which shows that this type of asthma can be developed on an experimental basis by exposing animals to single allergens with the help of adjuvants.[16]

It is important to distinguish here between the potential role of allergens as causes of atopic wheezing and their role in triggering attacks in individuals who are exposed and sensitized to these allergens. The latter is indisputable, and a large body of literature has convincingly shown that careful avoidance of certain exposures is associated with some symptom relief.[17-19] However, this in no way proves that these allergens are, in all such cases, the original cause of the disease.

The belief that allergens cause asthma has had very important consequences from the point of view of prevention strategies for the disease. For example, the most frequent allergens associated with asthma in coastal regions are *Dermatophagoides farinae* or *D. pteronyssinus*, which are microscopic mites present in house dust that require a significant degree of humidity to survive. For years, an entrenched belief was that house dust mites caused asthma and, therefore, prevention of the disease implied, as a crucial step, avoidance of exposure to dust mites.[20]

Recent observational, longitudinal studies have seriously challenged this concept. One such study followed children from the early school years up to late adolescence in

Dunedin, New Zealand.[21] One very important finding was that children who had persistent asthma symptoms during childhood became sensitized to different groups of allergens, unlike those observed among children who developed allergic rhinitis but not asthma. While the former showed, as a group, much more tendency to have positive skin-test reactions against house dust mites and pets, children with allergic rhinitis only were much more likely to be sensitized preferentially against seasonal allergens such as pollens.[22] If the 'allergic' theory of asthma were correct, it is difficult to understand why certain antigens should be more asthmogenic than others. Efforts have been made to try to identify some physical (smaller size and thus more penetration into the lower airway?) or biological (enzymatic properties that allow the allergen to penetrate the epithelial barrier?) characteristic of asthmogenic allergens, but the results have been disappointing and no such common property has yet been found. Perhaps the only shared characteristic of these asthma-related allergens is that they are invariably perennial: exposure occurs year round, frequently indoors,[23] and thus inevitably during the first years of life. We will return to this issue later in this chapter.

Perhaps the most convincing evidence against the traditional approach to understanding the pathogenesis of atopic wheezing was provided by a longitudinal study in which exposure to house dust mites in homes was assessed in a large number of children enrolled at birth in several cities in Germany.[24] The hypothesis was that if asthma is caused by house dust mites, individuals more heavily exposed to mites in their homes during the first years of life would be at higher risk for both allergic sensitization to mites and for the development of asthma. As expected, when these children were studied at 7 years of age, a strong association was found between incidence of asthma and incidence of sensitization to house dust mites at that age. Similarly, a strong association was found between the level of exposure to house dust mites in the homes during the first year of life and the likelihood of becoming sensitized to these acarids. Surprisingly, however, no association was found between exposure to house dust mite during the first years of life and the subsequent development of asthma (Figure 3.2).

The most plausible explanation for this finding is that the mechanisms by which individuals who will develop asthma are sensitized against house dust mites are different from those by which individuals who will not develop asthma become sensitized to the same allergens. In the former case, there is really no threshold for sensitization and most individuals can become sensitized with a very low level of exposure. Among subjects who will not become asthmatics, on the other hand, sensitization follows a dose–response relationship. Of great interest in this regard are studies performed in the island of Tristan da Cunha.[25] This island, located in the Atlantic midway between Africa and South America, is inhabited by a few hundred, quite heavily inbred persons with a very high prevalence of asthma, which was probably inherited from several of the few, very first colonizers of the island. Cats were exterminated from Tristan de Cunha 20 years ago and, in spite of this, 12.5% of individuals born after that event are allergic to cat. Thus, in an environment at high genetic risk for asthma, sensitization to allergens occurs at extremely low levels of exposure, much lower apparently than those needed to sensitize persons who are not predisposed to asthma.

The above discussion does not deny the possibility that individuals who become sensitized by the non-asthmatic, dose–response mechanism may also develop asthma-like

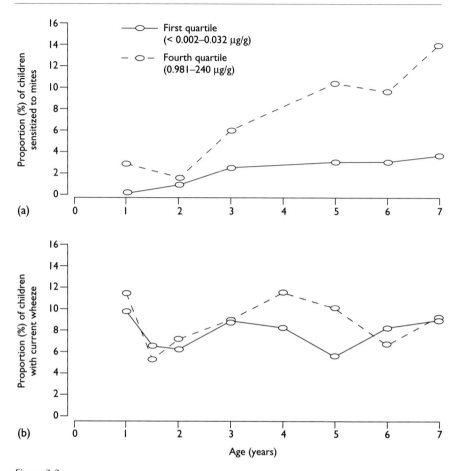

Figure 3.2

Association of exposure to house dust mites during the first year of life to (a) sensitization to house dust mites and (b) frequency of current wheezing, between the ages of 1 and 7. (From Lau et al[24] with permission from Elsevier).

symptoms later. As stated earlier, high levels of exposure to allergens may trigger asthma symptoms in susceptible individuals who can be sensitized only to these allergens. However, if this particular sensitization mechanism were the most frequent one in atopic wheezing of the early school years, a dose–response effect would have been observed between exposure to house dust mites and asthma risk in the German study, and that was not the case.

Different allergens, same asthma

The lack of a dose–response relationship between exposure to house dust mites and development of atopic wheezing challenges the concept that the former is the true cause of the latter. However, this is not the only evidence against this hypothesis. In fact, if it were correct, individuals raised in areas where, for example, house dust mites are not present in the environment should be at a much lower risk of developing atopic wheezing. Several studies have shown that this is not the case. In inland regions of both Australia and the USA (Arizona), where mites are very infrequently isolated from house dust due to the dry environment, asthma is as frequent as in the coastal regions.[26,27] In these desert-type environments, molds such as *Alternaria* appear to take the place of house dust mites, as sensitization to these allergens is most strongly associated with asthma. Several studies have shown that, in the inner cities of metropolitan areas of the USA, positive skin tests against cockroaches are the most prevalent form of sensitization observed in children with asthma.[28] Of particular interest regarding this same issue are the studies of prevalence of asthma and allergic sensitization in Northern Sweden.[29] In these barren lands, exposure to the allergens that are most frequently associated with atopic wheezing in other areas of the world is extremely low. However, prevalence of asthma is not different from that observed in Stockholm and other Swedish cities. In these areas, there is a strong association between sensitization to pets and asthma symptoms among schoolchildren, but the number of children with asthma who appear not to be sensitized against any of the usual allergens is very high. One could suspect that this is a form of non-atopic wheezing (see Chapter 1), but, interestingly, these same children have much higher levels of circulating IgE levels than those without asthma. The most likely explanation for this finding is that, in the almost complete absence of parasitic infestation in Northern Sweden, many of the aeroallergens that elicit IgE-mediated responses, and thus increase total serum IgE in these children with atopic asthma, have not even been identified.

Differences between early and late sensitization

Moreover, if atopic wheezing were caused by exposure and sensitization to a specific allergen, then the age at which this sensitization occurred would be irrelevant: the risk for the subsequent development of asthma should be the same, whatever the age at which sensitization first developed. Recent longitudinal studies show that the contrary is true. In coastal Australia, for example, children who became sensitized to house dust mites before the age of 8 were almost invariably also sensitized when re-tested at the age of 12, and had a very high risk of having asthma and persistent BHR.[30] However, among Australian children who were not sensitized by the age of 8 but who became sensitized thereafter, the risk of having persistent asthma symptoms and BHR was as low as that observed among those who were never sensitized. Very similar results were reported in a longer prospective study from the USA in which skin-test reactivity was measured repeatedly during childhood.[31] Children who were skin-test positive before the age of 8 were much more likely to have persistent wheezing symptoms than those who were sensitized after the age of 8. However, this study added an interesting twist: when children were tested a third time some years after the second test, those who were skin-test positive at the first test (before the age of 8) were much more likely to have persistent sensitization at the third test than those who became sensitized at the second test. Thus, late sensitization is not only not associated with significantly increased asthma risk, but it is also much more likely to remit, probably because the development of immunologic tolerance, which is a rare phenomenon among children who are sensitized against aeroallergens in early life, is much more frequent in those sensitized late in life.

It is interesting that the Australian study, which showed that early sensitization to house dust mites was associated with higher risk for asthma, was replicated in Tucson, Arizona.[32] In the Tucson study, however, house dust mites were not the incriminated allergen; it was early sensitization to *Alternaria* that was much more strongly associated with asthma than late sensitization to this same allergen.

Development of IFN-γ responses and atopic wheezing

The most reasonable explanation for all of these findings is that the most common form of atopic wheezing is not caused by sensitization to any specific allergen. More likely, subjects who are susceptible to developing asthma have an alteration in their immune system that predisposes them to produce IgE-type responses against many different asthma-related allergens that they encounter, especially during the first years of their life. In other words, it is quite likely (although not proven, and certainly very difficult to ever prove) that atopic wheezers sensitized to house dust mites in coastal regions would have been atopic wheezers sensitized to *Alternaria* in inland desert regions!

The nature of this alteration in immune development has not been completely eluci-dated. However, several lines of evidence suggest that a crucial factor is the maturation of the capacity to produce IFN-γ by immune cells during the first years of life. It is now well established that newborns have a global downregulation of cellular immune responses.[33,34] When experimentally stimulated, responses elicited in antigen-presenting cells as well as those by different types of T-cells are globally diminished. For example, both the production of those cytokines that are characteristic of helper T-cells (Th) type 1 (IFN-γ, IL-2 etc), as well as those that are characteristic of Th-2 (IL-4, IL-13 etc), are markedly decreased at birth. IL-10 is the only cytokine that, in response to non-specific stimuli, is produced by peripheral blood mononuclear cells during the newborn period in quantities that are similar to those observed in adults. It is of interest that IL-10 is a global downregulator of immune responses, and it is possible that this selec-tive normal production of IL-10 may play a role in the downregulation of the produc-tion of all other cytokines.

Although, as stated, immaturity of the immune system is global in newborns and neonates, production of Th-1 cytokines, and especially that of IFN-γ, is particularly depressed. Therefore, in the Th-1/Th-2 balance, newborns and neonate responses are skewed in favor of the Th-2 responses. There is naturally a distribution of such imbal-ances, with individuals whose parents are atopic having the highest prevalence of responses that are skewed against those of the Th-1 type.[35,36]

It is now also well established that the normal balance of Th-1/Th-2 responses is developmentally regulated and that it is usually established by the third year of life in all children with normal immune systems, including those with early atopy.[37] However, individuals who will go on to become sensitized against those allergens that are most strongly associated with asthma (i.e. *Alternaria* in the desert regions), show a marked delay in the development of IFN-γ responses during the first to second years of life.[38] By the end of the third year of life, however, these responses have caught up with those of

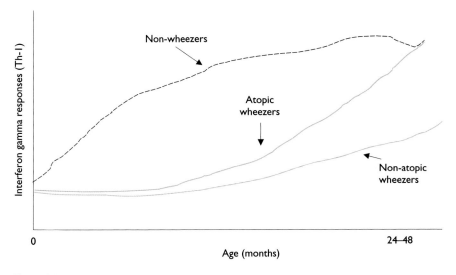

Figure 3.3

Association between interferon gamma (IFN-γ) responses and atopic and non-atopic wheezing during the first years of life. The figure has been drawn based on several different studies and should not be read as the result of a single, comprehensive study.

children who will not become sensitized to local aeroallergens (Figure 3.3). It is interesting to observe that a delay in the maturation of IFN-γ responses is often observed years before any evidence of sensitization against asthma-related aeroallergens is detectable by either skin-test or serum assays. Moreover, in most children who will go on to become atopic wheezers, wheezing episodes begin before any demonstrable evidence of allergic sensitization. This suggests that the immune factors that determine wheezing in these children are not the consequence of an IgE response occurring in their airways, at least not during the first stages of the disease. This concept is very important because once again it supports the hypothesis that, at least in this form of atopic asthma, sensitization to specific aeroallergens is not causally related to the disease.

TOWARDS A UNIFIED THEORY OF THE BEGINNINGS OF WHEEZING DISORDERS

IFN-γ responses in non-atopic and atopic wheezers

If allergens do not appear to be the direct cause of atopic wheezing, at least in its very first stages, the question that remains unanswered is what are the determinants of wheezing in these infants and young children. As has been stated earlier, atopic and non-atopic wheezing are clinically indistinguishable in early life, and the main triggers of wheezing episodes in both groups are viral infections. In a previous section, evidence was also presented suggesting that, much like atopic wheezers, non-atopic wheezers have diminished IFN-γ responses by PBMC when compared with children without a history of wheezing. Available data also suggest, however, that atopic wheezers have evidence of increased IL-4 responses by PBMC and of eosinophilic inflammation in the airways,[1,7] much like older children and adults with atopic asthma. This raises interesting and important questions: is the alteration in IFN-γ responses the same for both atopic and non-atopic wheezers? Is there, therefore, a common pathogenesis to both forms of wheezing during early life, associated with an alteration in immune responses to viruses? We do not have answers to these crucial questions at the present time. One potential scenario is that, although both forms of wheezing are associated with low IFN-γ responses and with altered immune reactivity to viruses, the cells responsible for these alterations may be different, thus giving rise to different biological consequences in both forms. Another scenario is that both atopic and non-atopic forms of wheezing effectively start as the same disease, caused by the same basic alteration. However, the presence of low IFN-γ responses would further predispose to the development of low-dose sensitization to aeroallergens only among atopic wheezers, because of an added predisposition to developing Th-2 responses in the latter, independent of the alteration in IFN-γ responses observed in both groups. In this second scenario, the alteration in IFN-γ responses would predispose both groups to viral wheezing in early life, but only atopic wheezers would have persistent wheezing due to the development of Th-2-mediated responses as a consequence of an additional genetic or developmental susceptibility that would not be present in non-atopic wheezers.

Unfortunately, there are currently no data to support or rule out either of these scenarios. However, if both forms of wheezing were initially associated with the same disease mechanism, observed secular trends should be similar for both forms. This hypothesis was indirectly tested by Kuehni et al.[39] These authors performed population surveys in 1990 and 1998 of the prevalence of respiratory symptoms in random samples of 1650 and 2600 children between the ages of 1 to 5 living in the county of Leicestershire, UK. Between 1990 and 1998, there was a significant increase in the prevalence of reported wheeze (16 to 29%), current wheeze (12 to 26%), diagnosis of asthma (11 to 19%), treatment for wheeze (15 to 26%) and admission for wheeze or other chest trouble (6 to 10%). The increase occurred both in children with viral wheeze (presumably non-atopic wheezers), 9 to 19%, and in those with the classic asthma pattern of wheezing with multiple triggers (presumably atopic wheezers in the nomenclature use in this book), 6 to 10%. All these changes were highly significant from a statistical point of view. The reasons why both forms could have increased during the past decades will be discussed later in this chapter. However, from the point of view of the arguments exposed here, the conclusions reached by Kuehni et al[39] appear cogent: what is determining these increases in the prevalence of asthma-like symptoms must be affecting a determinant of recurrent airway obstruction that is common to all forms of wheezing in early life.

Consequences of a Th-2 memory in the airways

The delay in the maturation of IFN-γ responses has very important consequences not only for reactivity against viruses but also in terms of the types of immune reactivity that is established against aeroallergens in children who are susceptible to become sensitized to these allergens, as described above. Experimental studies have demonstrated that the nature of the immune response that occurs at the time of the first encounter with these aeroallergens is an important determinant of the type of immune memory that will be established for future encounters with the same antigens. In other words, if the type of immune memory established at the first encounters is of Th-2, it is much more likely that similar responses will be elicited by subsequent encounters with the same antigen. In vitro studies have shown that IFN-γ has potent inhibitory effects on Th-2 responses, both in animal models and in experiments using human cells.[40] A delay in the maturation of IFN-γ responses may create the opportunity for certain antigens to be recognized with a Th-2 'lens' in certain, susceptible children. The consequence of this phenomenon could be that this type of immune response against these antigens is established very early during the process of formation of immunologic memory.

If the maturation of the immune system of the lung is delayed in the manner explained above, it is quite likely that the type of response elicited by many antigens that the susceptible neonate and infant is exposed to through the airways will be also skewed in favor of Th-2 responses. Indeed, this appears to be the case. For example, as part of the Tucson Children's longitudinal study, total serum IgE levels were measured before and after the first episode of LRI, at a mean of approximately 1 year of age.[41] Children who later became persistent wheezers (and especially atopic wheezers) showed significant increases in IgE at the time of the acute illness as compared with total serum IgE levels observed during the convalescent period. No such increases were observed among the children who would later be classified as transient wheezers. Although one possible explanation for this finding could be that children destined to become asthmatic respond with IgE specific for RSV,[42] this finding remains disputed.[43,44] More likely, acute infections may activate a polyclonal immune response to many antigens, and this response is likely to be skewed towards Th-2 in young infants predisposed to atopic wheezing.

These studies thus suggest that the delay in the maturation of Th-1 responses not only determines that children predisposed to atopic wheezing are more likely to become sensitized against aeroallergens in early life, but also suggests that these children have a global tendency to produce Th-2 responses against many antigens. This biased response system has very important consequences for lung growth and development, which we are only just beginning to understand. Very recent studies have convincingly shown that receptors for Th-2 cytokines are present not only in immune cells but also in fibroblasts and airway smooth muscle cells.[45,46] IL-4, but especially IL-13, act as growth factors for both these cell types.[47] Therefore, if the many antigens (including certain viruses) that we are inevitably exposed to during the first year of life, but especially those that are perennial in nature, elicit persistent Th-2-like responses in the airways, an undesired outcome could be an alteration in the normal process of structural lung development that occurs during these first years of life. Researchers interested in asthma often ignore the fact that the disease usually starts at a time when the lung is going through a normal process of growth that increases the size of the lungs and airways 5–10-fold in a 4–5 year interval. It is plausible to surmise that, in order to grow and at the same time maintain its efficient gas exchange functions, constant physiologic remodeling of the lung has to occur, and this process should be under the control of delicate developmental mechanisms. The potential for Th-2 cytokines to disrupt this process, as suggested by the latest work in this area, offers a cogent explanation for some of the epidemiologic data that we have reviewed in Chapter 1. Data currently available in which children were followed from birth up to the time in which they develop atopic wheezing suggest that this form of asthma is not associated with low levels of lung function measured shortly after birth. In fact, several longitudinal studies suggest that a significant proportion of the deficits in lung function observed in children and young adults with atopic asthma occur during the very early stages of the disease.[48] After the age of 7–10, lung function tracks markedly by levels of severity among asthmatics.[49,50] Therefore, it is most likely that a significant proportion of the losses in lung function and the state of BHR observed among atopic wheezers is acquired, and acquired early in the course of the disease (see Chapter 1). The finding that Th-2-like cytokines may act directly on smooth muscle cells and on the extracellular matrix suggests a cogent mechanism by which Th-2 bias in the airways may be responsible, at least in part, for the persistence of symptoms beyond the school years and for the alterations in lung function and BHR that have been observed in studies of the natural history of the disease.

Genetics of asthma and genetics of atopy

It is of interest to note here that the proposal that atopic wheezing is not caused by sensitization to any specific allergen is supported by genetic studies of asthma. The past five years have seen a flurry of reports of potential genetic determinants of asthma and allergies, and it is often difficult to make sense of results that are frequently not corroborated by other researchers performing apparently the same type of study. However, the most conspicuous result of these genetic studies is that inheritance of asthma is independent of that of specific markers of the atopic status, such as circulating IgE against allergens, skin-test reactivity to allergens etc.[51,52] These results thus suggest that there may be genetic determinants of atopic wheezing that are different from those of other forms of atopic disease, but that may be shared with those of non-atopic asthma. It is also possible that, together with genetic determinants that are common to both forms of wheezing, atopic and non-atopic, there are genetic determinants of allergy that are common to atopic wheezers and persons who have allergy but who do not wheeze. However, as explained earlier, it appears that the process by which children who develop atopic wheezing become sensitized to aeroallergens is different from that present in children who become sensitized to these same allergens but do not wheeze. This suggests that the genetics of these two forms of sensitization may also be different. Unfortunately, none of the genetic studies of allergies or asthma currently available have tested the hypotheses that different forms of allergic sensitization may have different hereditary bases, and that there may be common genetic determinants to atopic and non-atopic forms of wheezing in early life.

Environmental factors that regulate the development of INF-γ responses

If the explanations provided in the previous paragraphs are corroborated in future studies, it is plausible to surmise that the genetic and environmental factors that determine the maturation of IFN-γ responses early in life should play an important role in the development of both non-atopic and atopic forms of wheezing. These factors are only now beginning to be understood, and epidemiological studies have offered significant new clues. Perhaps the most tantalizing discovery about the epidemiology of asthma over the past 20 years is the observation that, in several different locales, exposure to domestic animals, to other children at home or in day care, or to animals on farms,[53–56] modifies the risk of having wheezing and sensitization to asthma-associated aeroallergens. The associations are not simple, straightforward and unidirectional. For example, exposure to other children in day care or to older siblings at home during the first year of life not only does not prevent non-atopic wheezing or transient wheezing, but may even be a risk factor for these conditions, whilst this same exposure has been shown to significantly decrease the likelihood of developing atopic wheezing during the school years. Conversely, exposure to animals on farms, and dogs and cats appears to consistently decrease the risk of both atopic and non-atopic wheezing in those studies in which such an effect was found.

Particularly relevant to this discussion is the fact that these exposures exert their preventive effects if they occur during the first years of life, and especially during infancy. This supports the contention that there is a critical period early in life (see Figure 3.3) during which the development of the immune response system requires certain environmental signals that trigger precoded maturational mechanisms. The concept that environmental signals are necessary for the different steps of the normal maturation of an organ system to occur in a timely manner, and that disruption of these signals may cause long-term sequelae, is not new. The importance of light exposure for the development of the retina and the visual cortex was probably the first such process to be disentangled almost 50 years ago, and similar findings have been made for other organ systems such as hearing, body balance etc. In the case of the immune system, the epidemiologic studies quoted above suggest that some factor common to day care, farms and pets, or perhaps different environmental factors for these three exposures, could regulate the development of immune responsiveness associated with asthma and allergies.

One potential common factor to all of the above exposures could be an increased exposure to microbial products. Indeed, children exposed to other children have a higher incidence of infections, especially viral but also bacterial, whereas those raised around pets and on animal farms have been shown to be more exposed to bacterial products such as endotoxin.[57,58] Endotoxin is a component of the cell walls of Gramnegative bacteria. Its main biologically active component is called lipopolysaccharide (LPS). LPS is a member of a family of so-called pathogen-associated molecular patterns (PAMP) that are present in the cell surface of most bacteria.[59] PAMP are invariably part of molecular systems that are crucial for bacterial survival, and these molecular systems are not encoded in the genome of eucaryotes. Probably because of these characteristics, PAMP have been selected through evolution as the signals of danger for the innate immune system. This system uses these signals to identify potential pathogens and to trigger the initial steps of the immune response. For this purpose, very ancient proteins, called Toll-like receptors (TLR), in acknowledgment of their homology with a similar protein first found in *Drosophila* called Toll, are encoded in the genomes of all studied vertebrates. These proteins recognize certain physico-biochemical patterns uniquely present in microbial PAMP, thus their common name, pattern recognition receptors (PRR). To date, it has been established, for example, that LPS is the ligand for TLR4, and that TLR4 requires several other molecules in order to process LPS, including a protein present both in the surface of antigen-presenting cells and in circulation called CD14 (see below). TLR2, on the other hand, is the receptor for PAMP from Gram-positive bacteria, such as peptidoglycan and lipoteichoic acid as well as for signals from *Mycobacteria* (e.g. lipoarabinomannams) and even for the respiratory syncytial virus, whereas TLR9 recognizes very specific nucleotide sequences (called CpGs) that are only present in bacterial DNA. PRR are present on the surface of many cells of the innate immune system, especially of antigen-presenting cells such as dendritic cells and macrophages, that are very abundant both in the lumen and in the walls of the airways. When stimulated by PAMP, PRR trigger signal transduction mechanisms in the cells that ultimately give way to the production of cytokines such as TNF-α, IL-12 and IL-10. These cytokines, on the one hand, attract other innate immunity cells that initiate the response to the invader and, on the other hand, act on Th cells to orient their responses either towards Th-1 or Th-2.

Of special importance in clarifying the nature of these environmental factors were the findings regarding the protective effect that living in farming communities in Canada[60] and Europe[61] has against atopic and non-atopic wheezing. The gist of these studies is simple: children raised in rural communities were divided into two groups. First, those raised on farms and second those raised in small towns in the same rural communities but away from farms. The results were very consistent: those raised on farms had markedly less risk of having non-atopic wheezing, atopic wheezing and sensitization to asthma-related allergens than those raised in towns. But these studies have an additional merit in that they allowed a more thorough assessment of the timing and specificity of exposures that could potentially explain the findings. An important discovery was that it was not a low socioeconomic condition that explained the results, because farmers had a very good standard of living in the European studies which were performed in Austria, Switzerland and Germany. A more detailed analysis showed that it was children raised close to animal farms who were at the lowest risk. Moreover, those infants whose parents fed them with unpasteurized farm milk during the first year of life or who were taken to the animal barns daily and for prolonged periods of time (usually by their mothers eager to milk their cows) were at the lowest risk for having both atopic and non-atopic wheezing during the school years.[55] This suggested that perhaps contact with animal products could be the protective factor for all forms of wheezing. In order to determine what these products could be, dust samples from both the homes and the stables were screened for several potential antigens and other substances. The most consistent finding was that endotoxin was abundantly more present in dust collected from farmers' homes and stables than from homes from town dwellers.[58]

Results of the studies in farm, day-care and pet-exposed children therefore suggested that endotoxin, or some other bacterial product that persons exposed to endotoxin could be co-exposed to, triggered maturational processes that enhanced the early development IFN-γ responses. This hypothesis was supported by the demonstration that infants and young children who are more heavily exposed to house dust endotoxin are more likely to develop stronger IFN-γ responses during the first year of life and less likely to become sensitized to allergens than those who are not as heavily exposed to endotoxin.[62] However, as explained earlier, young children who are heavily exposed to endotoxin in early life[12] and those exposed to other children[63] are more likely to have transient early wheezing. In the case of exposure to other children, a potential explanation is that these infants, together with being more exposed to bacterial products, are also more exposed to respiratory viruses, which makes them more likely to have transient wheezing episodes, at least while their IFN-γ responses are still immature.

Contradictory effects of endotoxin at different ages and at different times during the development of immune responses

That exposure to endotoxin may increase transient infant wheezing, however, appears to contradict the idea that this same exposure increases IFN-γ responses, and thus should protect against all forms of wheezing, if the hypothesis proposed herein is correct. Studies of experimental animals exposed to endotoxin during early life provided important clues that have helped us understand these apparent contradictions.[64] These studies showed that endotoxin has at least two effects on the lungs. On the one hand, it transiently increases bronchial responsiveness that is associated with recruitment of neutrophils and lymphocytes to the airway and, on the other hand, it transiently decreases IFN-γ concentrations in BAL fluid. Therefore, the short-term effect of endotoxin exposure on the developing immune system could be to increase severity of viral infections by decreasing acute IFN-γ responses, whereas its long-term effects could be to enhance the capacity of the immune system to develop these same IFN-γ responses, as suggested by Gereda et al.[62] These opposite effects of long- and short-term effects of bacterial products such as endotoxin on different forms of wheezing may depend on the diverse immune functions that are influenced by these bacterial products. On the one hand, these products may enhance immune responses mediated by activated alveolar macrophages, which is a cell that has the full complement of receptor components for endotoxin. By this mechanism, they may increase the likelihood of having wheezing episodes in early life, at a time when activated macrophages and a neutrophilic inflammation associated with it seems to predominate. On the other hand, chronic exposure to endotoxin at a crucial time during the development of the immune system may enhance the maturation of IFN-γ responses, which in turn may facilitate a more active response to viruses such as RSV and rhinoviruses, with less involvement of the lower airway. This dichotomy could explain the apparently paradoxical finding of more viral-associated, transient wheezing early in life and less wheezing (both atopic and non-atopic) later in life in children exposed to endotoxin.

Gene–environment interactions in the development of atopic and non-atopic wheezing

The identification of a specific group of proteins that act as receptors for environmental exposures, such as endotoxin, that may be associated with the prevention of atopic and non-atopic wheezing, offers a unique opportunity for studies of gene–environment interactions in the development of these two conditions. The reasoning behind this approach is straightforward: if genetic variants are present in the genes that encode for these proteins and these variants increase (or decrease) the expression of these proteins or their affinity for their ligands, then a logical consequence should be that these variants ought to be associated with atopic and non-atopic wheezing. In other words, the danger signals that promote IFN-γ responses should be modulated by the quality and quantity of the receptors for these signals present in the host. Studies of this type are only in their infancy because not all PRR have been exhaustively characterized, and therefore neither their genomic structure nor their PAMP ligands are always known. However, initial results obtained in studies of the best known of these receptor systems, that for LPS, are very indicative of the potential importance of these genetic variants.

As explained earlier, LPS interacts with TLR4 but requires the presence of a protein called CD14, which acts as the chaperone that presents it to TLR4. The gene for CD14 was the first to be screened for polymorphisms for the purpose of determining their potential role in the genetics of atopic wheezing and atopy.[65] These variants are usually associated with alternative nucleotides present at a certain position in the DNA sequence, resulting in two such sequences being present in the population. No variants that determined changes in the amino acid sequence of the CD14 protein were found in the coding region of the gene. However, one very frequent such variant (half of all chromosomes carried it) was found in the promoter region, i.e. in the area of the gene that regulates the rate of transcription and, therefore, the amount of protein that is ultimately synthesized (Figure 3.4). One of the alleles (T) for this variant was associated with higher levels of circulating CD14 and higher gene transcription rates than the other allele (C) (Figure 3.5).[65,66] That same T allele was found to be associated with

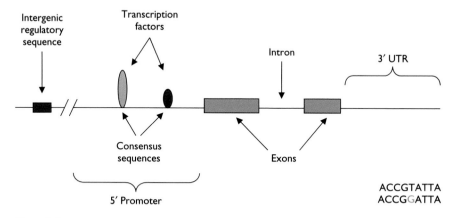

Figure 3.4

Potential locations of genetic variants within the structure of a gene and in surrounding DNA regions. Polymorphisms, including the most frequent form called single nucleotide polymorphisms (SNP, see lower right of figure for an example), can occur in many different areas of genes. For example, in exons (which contain the code for the amino acids), in introns located between the exons, in the 5′ promoter regions that regulate transcription rates through proteins called transcription factors, in the 3′ untranslated regions (3′ UTR) that regulate the stability of the mRNA, and in intergenic regulatory sequences that may regulate transcription of many different genes.

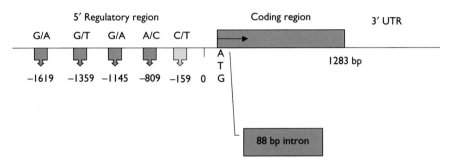

Figure 3.5

Structure of the human CD14 gene and location of the most important polymorphims found in this gene. It can be observed that most of these polymorphisms were located in the 5′ regulatory region. The polymorphism most often studied was that located at position −159 from the transcription start site.

lower serum IgE levels and/or with a lower number of positive skin tests in several (albeit not all) populations in which this association was studied.[67–69] However, none of the studies showed any association between this genetic variant and atopic asthma.

Interestingly, no association was found between variants in TLR4 and asthma in a genetic study performed in the same population enrolled in the Childhood Asthma Management Program (CAMP) study.[70] These results thus suggest that genetic variants in the CD14/TLR4 endotoxin receptor system may be important determinants of the risk for atopy but may play only a limited role in the genetics of wheezing. It is still premature to say, however, that this implies that exposure to their ligand, LPS, is an important prevention factor for atopy but not for wheezing. It is possible, for example, that the variants studied may not affect interactions between LPS and the receptor system in early life, when such interactions could probably be crucial for the development of wheezing, as described earlier. A lot of work is currently being done and new developments should be expected in the next few years.

IMMUNOLOGY OF WHEEZING AT THE BEGINNINGS OF LIFE: A COMPREHENSIVE VIEW

The inception of both atopic and non-atopic wheezing is the result of a complex set of interactions between genetic predisposition, environmental exposures and patterns of development of both immune responses and lung and airway systems (Figure 3.6). Persistence into the first years of life of the low IFN-γ responses that are characteristic of newborns predisposes infants to wheezing episodes during viral infections. The most important determinant of the maturation of IFN-γ responses is exposure to microbial products, which may, however, increase the likelihood of transient wheezing. In those children who do not have a genetic predisposition for allergies, non-atopic wheezing may persist as long as the deficit in IFN-γ responses persist, usually into the school years. If the child has a genetic predisposition for the development of Th-2 responses, low IFN-γ responses will also predispose the child to the development of early allergic

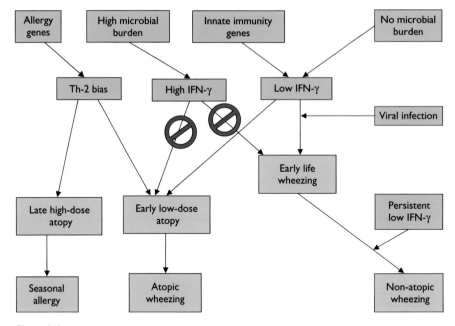

Figure 3.6

Proposed interaction between allergy-related risk factors and asthma-related risk factors in determining the development of different forms of wheezing and respiratory allergy during the first years of life. For a full explanation of the figure please consult the text.

sensitization at very low doses of allergen exposure during a crucial window of opportunity, or a critical period of postnatal life in which the nature of these responses is established. As a consequence, these individuals are more likely to develop Th-2 responses against many antigens, initially mainly against foods (see Chapter 1), but not much later against antigens that the subject is exposed to through the respiratory system. This is likely to create in the airways a local milieu in which Th-2 cytokines, acting as growth factors for airway smooth muscle cells and for the extracellular matrix, interfere with lung development and the regulation of airway tone, at a time of rapid lung and airway growth. One is tempted to speculate that the reason why patients with chronic atopic asthma are usually sensitized against perennial aeroallergens is because these allergens are the most likely to create a persistent Th-2 milieu in the airways. Likewise, the most severe subjects with atopic asthma are those sensitized against many allergens and this may also be a factor determining increased exposure of the airways to Th-2 cytokines. The final result is the combination of low lung function, BHR and altered responses to many environmental stimuli that are characteristic of the disease.

As stated earlier, this scenario does not certainly deny the possibility that atopic wheezing may also be the result of a process similar to that usually present in allergic rhinitis, in which sensitization to a single allergen (usually pollens) determines acute symptoms that respond well to elimination of the causative exposure or to immune therapy for that single culprit. However, in most persistent atopic wheezers the mechanism of disease is much more complex and global, and avoidance of single exposures may be helpful but seldom eliminates symptoms.

REFERENCES

1. Stevenson EC, Turner G, Heaney LG et al. Bronchoalveolar lavage findings suggest two different forms of childhood asthma. *Clin Exp Allergy* 1997; **27**: 1027–35.

2. Marguet C, Jouen-Boedes F, Dean TP, Warner JO. Bronchoalveolar cell profiles in children with asthma, infantile wheeze, chronic cough, or cystic fibrosis. *Am J Resp Crit Care Med* 1999; **159**: 1533–40.

3. Le Bourgeois M, Goncalves M, Le Clainche et al. Bronchoalveolar cells in children < 3 years old with severe recurrent wheezing. *Chest* 2002; **122**: 761–3.

4. Krawiec ME, Westcott JY, Chu HW et al. Persistent wheezing in very strong young children is associated with lower respiratory inflammation. *Am J Resp Crit Care Med* 2001; **163**: 1290–1.

5. Azevedo I, de Blic J, Dumarey CH et al. Increased spontaneous release of tumour necrosis factor-alpha by alveolar macrophages from wheezy infants. *Eur Resp J* 1997; **10**: 1767–73.

6. Azevedo I, de Blie J, Vargaftig BB et al. Increased eosinophil cationic protein levels in bronchoalveolar lavage from wheezy infants. *Pediatr Allergy Immunol* 2001; **12**: 65–72.

7. Koning H, Neijens HJ, Baert MR et al. T cell subsets and cytokines in allergic and non-allergic children I. Analysis of IL-4, IFN-gamma and IL-13 mRNA expression and protein production. *Cytokine* 1997; **9**: 416–26.

8. Leech SC, Price JF, Holmes BJ, Kemeny DM. Nonatopic wheezy children have reduced interferon-gamma. *Allergy* 2000; **55**: 74–8.

9. Bont L, Heijnen CJ, Kavelaars A et al. Monocyte IL-10 production during respiratory syncytial virus bronchiolitis is associated with recurrent wheezing in a one-year follow-up study. *Am J Resp Crit Care Med* 2000; **161**: 1518–23.

10. Makela MJ, Kanehiro A, Dakhama A et al. The failure of interleukin-10-deficient mice to develop airway hyperresponsiveness is overcome by respiratory syncytial virus infection in allergen-sensitized/challenged mice. *Am J Resp Crit Care Med* 2002; **165**: 824–31.

11. Grunstein MM, Hakonarson H, Leiter J et al. Autocrine signaling by IL-10 mediates altered responsiveness of atopic sensitized airway smooth muscle. *Am J Physiol Lung Cell Molec Physiol* 2001; **281**: L1130–7.

12. Litonjua AA, Milton DK, Celedon JC et al. A longitudinal analysis of wheezing in young children: the independent effects of early life exposure to house dust endotoxin, allergens, and pets. *J Allergy Clin Immunol* 2002; **110**: 736–42.

13. Sears MR. Evolution of asthma through childhood. *Clin Exp Allergy* 1998; **28** (**Suppl 5**): 82–9.

14. Wolfe R, Carlin JB, Oswald H et al. Association between allergy and asthma from childhood to middle adulthood in an Australian cohort study. *Am J Resp Crit Care Med* 2000; **162**: 2177–81.

15. Sears MR. Consequences of long-term inflammation. The natural history of asthma. *Clin Chest Med* 2000; **21**: 315–29.

16. Leong KP, Huston DP. Understanding the pathogenesis of allergic asthma using mouse models. *Ann Allergy Asthma Immunol* 2001; **87**: 96–109.

17. Downs SH, Mitakakis TZ, Marks GB et al. Clinical importance of *Alternaria* exposure in children. *Am J Crit Care Med* 2001; **164**: 455–9.

18. Strachan DP. House dust mite allergen avoidance in asthma. Benefits unproved but not yet excluded. *Br Med J* 1998; **317**: 1096–7.

19. Murray CS, Woodcock A, Custovic A. The role of indoor allergen exposure in the development of sensitization and asthma. *Curr Opin Allergy Clin Immunol* 2001; 1: 407–12.

20. Peat J, Bjorksten B. Primary and secondary prevention of allergic asthma. *Eur Resp J* 1998; 27: 28S–34S.

21. Sears MR, Jones DT, Silva PA et al. Asthma in seven year old children: a report from the Dunedin Multidisciplinary Child Development Study. *NZ Med J* 1982; 98: 533–6.

22. Sears MR, Burrows B, Flannery EM et al. Atopy in childhood. I. Gender and allergen related risks for development of hay fever and asthma. *Clin Exp Allergy* 1993; 23: 941–8.

23. Platts-Mills TA, Blumenthal K, Perzanowski M, Woodfolk JA. Determinants of clinical allergic disease. The relevance of indoor allergens to the increase in asthma. *Am J Crit Care Med* 2000; 162: S128–S133.

24. Lau S, Illi S, Sommerfeld C et al. Early exposure to house-dust mite and cat allergens and development of childhood asthma: a cohort study. *Lancet* 2000; 356: 1392–7.

25. Chan-Yeung M, McClean PA Sandell PR et al. Sensitization to cat without direct exposure to cats. *Clin Exp Allergy* 1999; 29: 762–5.

26. Halonen M, Stern DA, Wright AL et al. *Alternaria* as a major allergen for asthma in children raised in a desert environment. *Am J Resp Crit Care Med* 1997; 155: 1356–61.

27. Peat JK, Toelle BG, Gray EJ et al. Prevalence and severity of childhood asthma and allergic sensitisation in seven climatic regions of New South Wales. *Med J Aust* 1995; 163: 22–6.

28. Alp H, Yu BH, Grant EN et al. Cockroach allergy appears early in life in inner-city children with recurrent wheezing. *Ann Allergy Asthma Immunol* 2001; 86: 514.

29. Perzanowski MS, Ronmark E, Nold B et al. Relevance of allergens from cats and dogs to asthma in the northernmost province of Sweden: schools as a major site of exposure. *J Allergy Clin Immunol* 1999; 103: 1018–24.

30. Peat JK, Salome CM, Woolcock AJ. Longitudinal changes in atopy during a 4-year period: relation to bronchial hyperresponsiveness and respiratory symptoms in a population sample of Australian schoolchildren. *J Allergy Clin Immunol* 1990; 85: 65–74.

31. Sherrill D, Stein R, Kurzius-Spencer M, Martinez F. On early sensitization to allergens and development of respiratory symptoms. *Clin Exp Allergy* 1999; 29: 905–11.

32. Halonen M, Stern DA, Lohman IC, et al. Two subphenotypes of childhood asthma that differ in maternal and paternal influences on asthma risk. *Am J Resp Crit Care Med* 1999; 160: 564–70.

33. Wilson CB, Phenix L, Weaver WM et al. Ontogeny of T lymphocyte function in the neonate. *Am J Reprod Immunol* 1992; 28: 132–5.

34. Jones CA, Warner JO. Regulating a regulator: IFNgamma production by the neonate. *Clin Exp Allergy* 1999; 29: 865–8.

35. Miles EA, Warner JA, Lane AC et al. Altered T lymphocyte phenotype at birth in babies born to atopic parents. *Pediatr Allergy Immunol* 1994; 5: 202–8.

36. Martinez FD, Stern DA, Wright AL et al. Association of interleukin-2 and interferon-gamma production by blood mononuclear cells in infancy with parental allergy skin tests and with subsequent development of atopy. *J Allergy Clin Immunol* 1995; 96: 652–60.

37. Holt PG, Rudin A, Macaubas C et al. Development of immunologic memory against tetanus toxoid and pertactin antigens from the diphtheria–tetanus–pertussis vaccine in atopic versus nonatopic children. *J Allergy Clin Immunol* 2000; 105: 1117–22.

38. Martinez FD, Holt PG. Role of microbial burden in aetiology of allergy and asthma. *Lancet* 1999; 354 (**Suppl 2**): SII 12–15.

39. Kuehni CE, Davis A, Brooke AM, Silverman M. Are all wheezing disorders

in very young (preschool) children increasing in prevalence? *Lancet* 2001; **357**: 1821–5. (Erratum appears in *Lancet* 2001; **358**: 846.)

40. Romagnani S. T-cell responses in allergy and asthma. *Curr Opin Allergy Clin Immunol* 2001; **1**: 73–8.

41. Martinez FD, Stern DA, Wright AL et al. Differential immune responses to acute lower respiratory illness in early life by subsequent development of persistent wheezing and asthma. *J Allergy Clin Immunol* 1998; **102**: 915–20.

42. Welliver RC, Duffy L. The relationship of RSV-specific immunoglobulin E antibody responses in infancy, recurrent wheezing, and pulmonary function at age 7–8 years. *Pediatr Pulmonol* 1993; **15**: 19–27.

43. De Alarcon A, Walsh EE, Carper HT et al. Detection of IgA and IgG but not IgE antibody to respiratory syncytial virus in nasal washes and sera from infants with wheezing. *J Pediatr* 2001; **138**: 311–17.

44. Welliver RC, Ogra PL. RSV, IgE, and wheezing. *J Pediatr* 2001; **139**: 903–5.

45. Laporte JC, Moore PE, Baraldo S et al. Direct effects of interleukin-13 on signaling pathways for physiological responses in cultured human airway smooth muscle cells. *Am J Resp Crit Care Med* 2001; **164**: 141–8.

46. Doucet C, Brouty-Boye D, Pottin-Clemenceau C et al. IL-4 and IL-13 specifically increase adhesion molecule and inflammatory cytokine expression in human lung fibroblasts. *Int Immunol* 1998; **10**: 1421–33.

47. Doucet C, Brouty-Boye D, Pottin-Clemenceau C et al. Interleukin (IL)-4 and IL-13 act on human lung fibroblasts. Implication in asthma. *J Clin Invest* 1998; **101**: 2129–39.

48. Martinez FD. Present and future treatment of asthma in infants and young children. *J Allergy Clin Immunol* 1999; **104**: 169–74.

49. Oswald H, Phelan PD, Lanigan A et al. Childhood asthma and lung function in mid-adult life. *Pediatr Pulmonol* 1997; **23**: 14–20.

50. Rasmussen F, Taylor DR, Flannery EM et al. Risk factors for airway remodeling in asthma manifested by a low post-bronchodilator FEV1/vital capacity ratio: a longitudinal population study from childhood to adulthood. *Am J Resp Crit Care Med* 2002; **165**: 1480–8.

51. Los H, Koppelman GH, Postma DS. The importance of genetic influences in asthma. *Euro Resp J* 1999; **14**: 1210–27.

52. Holberg CJ, Halonen M, Solomon S et al. Factor analysis of asthma and atopy traits shows 2 major components, one of which is linked to markers on chromosome 5q. *J Allergy Clin Immunol* 2001; **108**: 772–80.

53. Celedon JC, Litonjua AA, Ryan L et al. Exposure to cat allergen, maternal history of asthma, and wheezing in first 5 years of life. *Lancet* 2002; **360**: 781–2.

54. Holscher B, Frye C, Wichmann HE, Heinrich J. Exposure to pets and allergies in children. *Pediatr Allergy Immunol* 2002; **13**: 334–41.

55. Riedler J, Braun-Fahrlander C, Eder W et al. Exposure to farming in early life and development of asthma and allergy: a cross-sectional survey. *Lancet* 2001; **358**: 1129–33.

56. Ball TM, Castro-Rodriguez JA, Griffith KA et al. Siblings, day-care attendance, and the risk of asthma and wheezing during childhood. *N Engl J Med* 2000; **343**: 538–43.

57. Park JH, Spiegelman DL, Gold DR et al. Predictors of airborne endotoxin in the home. *Envir Health Perspec* 2001; **109**: 859–64.

58. Von Mutius E, Braun-Fahrlander C, Schierl R et al. Exposure to endotoxin or other bacterial components might protect against the development of atopy. *Clin Exp Allergy* 2000; **30**: 1230–4.

59. Armant MA, Fenton MJ. Toll-like receptors: a family of pattern-recognition receptors in mammals. *Genome Biol* 2002; **3**: Reviews3011.

60. Ernst P, Cormier Y. Relative scarcity of asthma and atopy among rural adolescents raised on a farm. *Am J Resp Crit Care Med* 2000; **161**: 1563–6.

61. von Mutius E. Environmental factors influencing the development and progression of pediatric asthma. *J Allergy Clin Immunol* 2002; **109**(Suppl 6): S525–32.

62. Gereda JE, Leung DYM, Thatayatikon A et al. Relation between house-dust endotoxin exposure, type 1 T-cell development, and allergen sensitization in infants at high risk of asthma. *Lancet* 2000; **355**: 1680–3.

63. Infante-Rivard C, Amre D, Gautrin D, Malo JL. Family size, day-care attendance, and breastfeeding in relation to the incidence of childhood asthma. *Am J Epidemiol* 2001; **153**: 653–8.

64. Cochran JR, Khan AM, Elidemir O et al. Influence of lipopolysaccharide exposure on airway function and allergic responses in developing mice. *Pediatr Pulmonol* 2002; **34**: 267–77.

65. Baldini M, Lohman IC, Halonen M et al. A polymorphism in the 5'-flanking region of the CD 14 gene is associated with circulating soluble CD14 levels and with total serum IgE. *Am J Resp Cell Molec Biol* 1999; **20**: 976–83.

66. LeVan TD, Bloom JW, Bailey TJ et al. A common single nucleotide polymorphism in the CD14 promoter decreases the affinity of Sp protein binding and enhances transcriptional activity. *J Immunol* 2001; **167**: 5838–44.

67. Koppelman GH, Reijmerink NE, Colin Stine O et al. Association of a promoter polymorphism of the CD14 gene and atopy. *Am J Resp Crit Care Med* 2001; **163**: 965–9.

68. Gao PS, Mao XQ, Baldini M et al. Serum total IgE levels and CD14 on chromosome 5q31. *Clin Genet* 1999; **56**: 164–5.

69. Ober C, Tsalenko A, Parry R, Cox NJ. A second-generation genomewide screen for asthma-susceptibility alleles in a founder population. *Am J Hum Genet* 2000; **67**: 1154–62.

70. Raby BA, Klimecki WT, Laprise C et al. Polymorphisms in toll-like receptor 4 are not associated with asthma or atopy-related phenotypes. *Am J Resp Crit Care Med* 2002; **166**: 1449–56.

4

Clinical features of the wheezy infant

INTRODUCTION

Who are the wheezy infants and preschool children?

Wheezing is a very common symptom in infants and preschool children. In a national survey in the USA some 27% of all children under 18 years of age incurring medical costs for asthma were in the 0–4 years age group.[1] As discussed more fully in Chapter 1, wheezing is reported in almost 50% of infants before 6 years of age in some surveys. In the USA, a prospective cohort study followed children to 6 years of age and it was found that approximately 20% of all infants had transient wheezing before 3 years of age, an additional 14% of infants had continued to wheeze until 6 years of age, and some 15% had begun to wheeze after 3 years and had continued until 6 years of age.[2] Similarly, Young et al[3] reported an incidence of wheezing of 50% in Australian infants in the first two years of life, but a lower incidence of about 29% was found in preschool children in the UK[4] and 17% by 6–7 years of age in Italy.[5] From Australia, Oddy et al[6] reported an incidence of wheezing lower respiratory tract illness of 25% in a cohort study, and of this cohort 18% were diagnosed as having asthma at 6 years of age. In prospective studies of unselected populations of infants who wheezed between the first and third years of life, as well as in those with respiratory syncytial virus (RSV) bronchiolitis in early infancy, some 30–40% or more will continue to wheeze over the next 2–4 years.[2,5,7–9] However, most infants with RSV bronchiolitis have a single attack of bronchiolitis from which they recover in a few days (Chapter 2).

There is considerable confusion over the nomenclature of wheezing diseases in very young children, partly due to uncertainty over the etiology. It must be emphasized that there are two important groups of wheezy infants and preschool children. The large majority are termed 'typical' and the minority 'atypical' wheezy infants and preschool children.

- The **typical** wheezy infant or preschool child has symptoms that usually begin during the first year or two of life which may continue into childhood. Some cases will have an atopic background, while in others there is a clear relationship to viral infections; however, none of these children have any other significant underlying disease.
- The **atypical** wheezy infant or preschool child has symptoms that may begin at any time but in whom the disease is neither due to atopy nor viral infections and can be life-threatening in some cases. This group includes infants with well-defined diseases such as cystic fibrosis (CF), primary ciliary dyskinesia and congenital pulmonary or cardiac anomalies.

55

Within the large group of typical wheezy infants or preschool children, recent epidemiologic research has indicated that there are at least three important and distinct subgroups. There are some infants and preschool children with an obvious personal or family background of atopic diseases, many, but not all, of whom will go on to develop classical childhood asthma – we have termed them atopic infants or preschool wheezers. Many other infants, probably the large majority, have no personal or family background of atopy or asthma and begin to wheeze probably as a result of viral infection – we have termed all these infants and preschool children non-atopic infants or preschool wheezers. As discussed more fully in Chapter 5, some of the non-atopic wheezy infants have rather low normal levels of lung function before ever starting to wheeze[10,11] and in these children it is likely that viral infections cause some transient mechanical obstruction of the airways. The wheezing attacks in such infants tend to be transient in the first few months of life. Other infants and preschool children may have recurrent wheezing for several months or years in response to viral infections, or even non-infectious stimuli, because an initial viral infection has damaged the airways and induced a type of bronchial hyperresponsiveness (BHR). Some of these viral-induced wheezy infants begin to wheeze during the first years of life and would be difficult to distinguish from the 'transient early wheezers' of Martinez et al,[2] while others would have begun later and would have been included in their 'late-onset wheezers'. To summarize, typical wheezy infants or preschool children are either transient early non-atopic wheezers, non-atopic (viral) wheezers or atopic wheezers.

In older children the incidence of established asthma varies from country to country, but in most of Europe, North America and Australasia the incidence is between 10 and 30% according to an International Study of Asthma and Allergies in Childhood (ISAAC) survey.[12] Most asthmatic children will have developed symptoms by about 6 years of age, with the onset of asthma in older children less common.[4,13,14] Since the large majority of asthmatic children are atopic,[12,15,16] it is reasonable to assume that these children would have come from the group of younger atopic wheezers, which implies that some 80% of wheezy infants and preschool children would have been in the non-atopic groups. It is probable that most non-atopic children wheeze in response to viral infections, especially with the RSV but also with other viruses. Einarsson et al[17] showed that three of the most common viral precipitants of asthma, RSV, parainfluenza virus and rhinovirus (RV), were able to stimulate cytokine interleukin (IL)-11 production and that this cytokine could be detected in the nasal secretions of children with viral infections. They also found that the presence of IL-11 correlated with clinically apparent wheezing and that IL-11 was a potent inducer of BHR to methacholine in the mouse lung. In a recent study in adult human volunteers, Mckean et al[18] showed that viral inoculation in both atopic and non-atopic subjects, but not in uninoculated controls, induced wheeze, chest tightness and shortness of breath, and progressive BHR, on days 2, 4 and 17 after inoculation. It has also been shown that the presence of RSV IgE in infants is related to later wheezing in childhood.[19]

HOW WELL DO PARENTS RECOGNIZE WHEEZING IN THEIR CHILDREN?

When attempting to understand what is troubling the infant or preschool child with noisy breathing the pediatrician is always at a disadvantage, since the history has to be taken from a third party, normally one or the other of the parents. It may be difficult, indeed impossible, to understand what the parent means when complaining that their child has wheezy or noisy breathing. Parents may not understand what the physician means by wheeze and may use alternative terms such as noisy breathing, difficult breathing, croupy breathing, cough or stridor. Snoring due to nasopharyngeal obstruction is common in preschool children with adenoid hypertrophy. Because allergic rhinitis is also common in atopic children, even in the preschool age group, it is possible that snoring from this cause may coexist with asthma in some children. In some languages there may not be a simple translation of the term wheeze and therefore it is important to try to understand as clearly as possible what the parent means. Attempts have been made to examine clinical descriptors such as wheeze and the reliability with which they are reported by parents or children. Cane et al[20] undertook a study to determine what the parents of wheezy children understood by wheeze. In a group of predominantly preschool children (median of 2.5 years of age) the agreement between the parents and the physician as to the presence of wheezing or asthma was only 45%. In a subsequent study, in which they showed parents video clips, only 59% correctly recognized wheezing.[21] Even when parents were trained to recognize wheezing, Lee et al[22] found that parents recognized obvious wheeze but when wheezing was faint it was only recognized in 68% of observations.

Typical versus atypical wheezing – a critical distinction

The symptoms that parents can observe in very young children are rather limited and common to a number of different disorders of the respiratory system. The usual complaints are of cough, noisy breathing, wheezing and respiratory distress, symptoms which may occur in widely differing conditions such as asthma, adenoid hypertrophy, foreign-body aspiration and congenital tracheomalacia. It often happens that by the time the child is brought to the pediatrician the symptom is no longer present, which makes the complaint even harder to evaluate given the problems with interpreting parental observations. Even when the infant or young child is still symptomatic when seen by the pediatrician, this does not necessarily resolve the issue, since several different diseases may present with an almost identical clinical picture of tachypnea, distress, hyperinflation and polyphonic, musical wheezing. As shown in Figure 4.1, a similar clinical picture of wheezing in infancy and early childhood may have a typical or atypical origin and within each of these two groups there are a number of different possible causes of the problem.

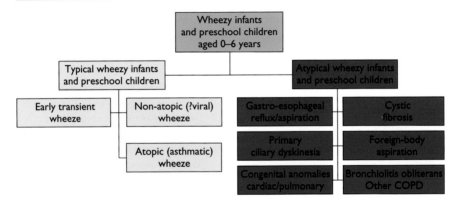

Figure 4.1

Schematic illustration of types of wheezy infants and preschool children. (COPD, Chronic obstructive pulmonary disease.)

CLINICAL FEATURES OF THE TYPICAL WHEEZY INFANT AND PRESCHOOL CHILD

We shall now consider some of the important clinical features and the management of the typical wheezy infant, in particular those features which should lead us to suspect that the problem may be atypical.

History

The typical wheezy infant may well have had a few attacks of wheeze before being brought to a specialist pediatrician for an expert opinion. Typical wheezing is characteristically very episodic at this age and infants and young children with typical wheezing should not have prolonged or continuous attacks. Chronic asthma simply does not occur in the typically wheezy infant or preschool child. The attacks last a few days and are separated by long symptom-free intervals. The duration and severity of the attacks are variable, and the child will often recover spontaneously without medical attention. There are a number of important points to be obtained from the history which help in evaluating the type of problem and the approach to management.

When did the child first develop wheezy or noisy breathing?

Acute viral bronchiolitis, usually due to infection with RSV, normally attacks infants in the 2–4 month age group and those who continue to wheeze after the attack will have begun to have symptoms at this age. Some 25% of children with asthma report their initial symptoms in the first year of life[14,23] and would be classified as atopic wheezy infants, but most asthmatic children start having overt symptoms rather later, usually between the ages of 2 and 6.[4,13,14] Children with wheezing due to bronchopulmonary dysplasia and similar conditions will normally have been born prematurely and have had respiratory problems very early on in life. Congenital anomalies of the airways, which can cause noisy breathing or wheezing, may present soon after birth, while other anomalies and other causes of wheezing, may present much later. Very early or very late onset of wheezing should raise the suspicion that the problem is atypical.

What has been the pattern of the attacks of wheeze or noisy breathing?

The typical wheezy child has attacks lasting a few days, with or without signs of an upper respiratory infection. The child will usually cough as well as wheeze and parents may only notice the cough. Frequently, symptoms are more troublesome at night but this is common to many conditions causing wheeze in infants. Once the attack has subsided the child is typically quite well until the next episode, which may occur after a number of weeks or even months. It is very important to be sure that there are these long symptom-free intervals because if the wheeze is continuous, or nearly continuous, then there is a much greater likelihood of a serious problem such as a congenital anomaly, CF or even an inhaled foreign body. Exercise is a potent trigger for wheezing in older asthmatic children but preschool children will rarely exercise hard enough or for long enough (5–6 minutes) to produce wheeze.[24] Nevertheless, if parents report that their child wheezes or coughs after running around or climbing stairs this should be taken as a possible sign that the problem is asthma. Since exercise-induced asthma is triggered by the heat and water loss which occurs because of the hyperventilation of exercise, it can also be triggered by vigorous crying or laughing, which are the preschool equivalents of hyperventilation-induced asthma.

How bad are the attacks?

Most wheezy infants and preschool children have a mild degree of airways obstruction which has very little effect on their normal activities. When the degree of obstruction is more severe the parents may notice that the child is breathing faster than normal; when even more severe, infants may have difficulty in feeding normally and preschool children may have difficulty in running about or even talking normally. Attacks severe enough to cause the child to become centrally cyanosed or to become apneic are very rare indeed. Because symptoms often occur during the night, even relatively mild wheezing can be perceived as serious by the parents and may well affect their quality of life.

Is there a personal or family background of atopic diseases or smoking?

Allergies are very common in the community and a family history should only be regarded as positive if it affects parents or siblings of the patient. Personal atopy such as infantile eczema is about twice as common and maternal asthma is more than twice as common[2] in infants with persistent or recurrent wheezing as compared to those with transient early wheezing.[25] In some societies there is a common belief that drinking cow's milk causes the infant to wheeze or produce sputum. While true milk allergy and lactose intolerance certainly do occur in infancy, they mainly produce gastrointestinal symptoms and it is rare for wheezing in infancy to be due to milk allergy.[26] When wheezing is due to true milk allergy, it is almost always accompanied by urticaria or other severe skin rashes. In a highly selected population of 32 children with milk allergy proven by challenge, cough or wheeze was present in 38%, and in 75% of these it was accompanied by urticaria with symptoms appearing within 10 minutes of ingesting milk.[27] Cigarette smoking is by far the most important environmental pollutant for infants and preschool children, but while parental, and especially maternal, smoking increases the likelihood of lower respiratory tract disorders in children it does not appear to distinguish between those with atopic and non-atopic wheezing.[2,3,28]

Physical examination

In the typical wheezy infant or preschool child the purpose of physical examination is to try to determine the origin of the noisy breathing and to exclude causes of wheeze or noisy breathing other than that due to the common type of atopic or non-atopic wheezing. In addition, the severity of the respiratory distress is assessed. Physical examination to determine the nature and severity of the wheeze is often problematic since many children may no longer be experiencing an attack when they come to be examined. Even if the child is symptomatic, the severity of the obstruction can vary markedly depending on the pattern of breathing, so the signs may fluctuate quite rapidly. Particular attention should be paid to a number of points in the examination.

General development

Traditionally, the common type of wheezy infant has been described as the 'fat, happy, wheezy baby', but there are little or no objective data to support this belief. In one study it was found that the early introduction of solids to the infant diet was associated with an increased probability of wheeze during childhood, and with increased percentage of body fat and weight.[29] If the infant is underweight, this could indicate failure to thrive, such as occurs in CF and certain other serious pulmonary or cardiac disorders. The common type of atopic or non-atopic recurrent wheezing should not cause the infant to be underweight. Infantile eczema, typically on the scalp or face, may indicate that the child is atopic.

Respiratory system

Unless there is some other underlying problem, the shape of the chest in the typical wheezy infant or preschool child should be normal and symmetrical. The findings on examination of the lungs obviously depend upon the state of the infant at the time and not infrequently the child is perfectly well by the time he/she reaches the physician. Care is needed not to mistake noisy breathing due to adenoid hypertrophy or laryngeal disease for wheezing originating in the intrapulmonary airways. During an attack, the signs include hyperinflation, prolonged expiration and generalized wheezing with or without subcostal retractions. In infants with milder obstruction the wheeze is only heard during expiration, or more correctly during late expiration. In general, as obstruction gets worse the wheeze is heard throughout expiration, and later on during inspiration as well. Wheeze is probably due to the fluttering of the walls of medium-sized airways,[30] which lie in the first 5–7 generations of branching of the airways (the trachea is generation 0), and is usually a musical, polyphonic sound, although sometimes it may be only monophonic. Provided that the sound occurs during expiration, monophonic wheezing is probably due to smaller airways obstruction. Care is needed with monophonic sounds which are only heard during inspiration as these are far more likely to originate in the larynx such as occurs in croup or congenital laryngeal stridor. Sounds which are low pitched or lack a musical characteristic, and especially if heard centrally rather than over the lung fields, may well be due to anomalies of the trachea or large airways such as tracheomalacia. In very severe obstruction it is claimed that the breath sounds may become so quiet that the wheeze is not audible – the silent chest – but in such infants other signs indicating severe distress should be obvious. Crackles (crepitations) are not typically heard in children with recurrent wheezing but are very common in the infant with acute viral bronchiolitis. However, the child with recurrent wheezing may develop expiratory crackles as well as wheeze during a moderate to severe exacerbation and such crackles do not necessarily indicate that the child has pneumonia. Coarse inspiratory and/or expiratory crackles indicate secretions in the large central airways or throat and are not of diagnostic importance for the wheezy infant. Central cyanosis is very uncommon except in the most severe attacks but parents often complain that the child has perioral cyanosis, the meaning of which is far from clear.

Evaluation of distress

The severity of the airways obstruction in the typical wheezy infant or preschool child has traditionally been evaluated by looking at a number of physical signs. These include the severity of wheezing, the effort needed for breathing as indicated by use of accessory muscles and retractions, the respiratory rate and the heart rate. In order to quantify these signs, various scoring methods have been developed, such as that of Tal et al[31] in which respiratory rate, wheezing intensity, circumoral or general cyanosis and use of accessory muscles were included. A more modern form of this score took age into account when scoring respiratory rate and used the concentration of supplementary oxygen needed in place of cyanosis.[32] In a recent study of wheezing in infants and preschool children we further developed the score in order to take account of the effect of age on both respiratory rate and heart rate (Table 4.1), and replaced the very indefinite signs of cyanosis or oxygen requirement with the objective measurement of oxygen saturation by pulse oximetry. The details of this scoring system are given in Table 4.2. In this system the maximum possible score is 15 and in our study of 31 wheezy infants and preschool children attending a hospital walk-in clinic, five scored ≤ 4, 21 scored 5–9 and five scored 10–11. If the child has received repeated doses of inhaled β_2-agonists the heart rate will be elevated and as a less useful index of the severity of obstruction.

Investigations

In the young child with recurrent episodes of wheezing and no unusual features in the history or physical examination, the number of investigations that are needed is quite limited. Unfortunately, there has been an increasing tendency over the years to perform

Table 4.1 Effect of age on scores used for respiratory rate and heart rate in wheezy infants and preschool children

Age (years)	Score = 0 Normal	Score = 1 Mildly elevated	Score = 2 Moderately elevated	Score = 3 Markedly elevated
Respiratory rate				
< 1	< 35	35–44	45–54	≥ 55
1–3	< 25	25–34	35–44	≥ 45
3–6	< 20	20–24	25–34	≥ 35
Heart rate				
< 1	< 140	140–159	160–179	≥ 180
1–3	< 120	120–134	135–159	≥ 160
3–6	< 100	100–109	110–129	≥ 130

Table 4.2 Scoring system for wheezy infants and preschool children

Score	0	1	2	3
Respiratory rate	Normal	Mildly elevated	Moderately elevated	Markedly elevated
Heart rate	Normal	Mildly elevated	Moderately elevated	Markedly elevated
Wheeze	None	End expiratory	Whole of expiration	Inspiratory and expiratory
Distress retractions	None	Mild	Moderate	Severe
Saturation	≥ 95%	92–94%	90–92%	< 90%

more and more investigations in such patients in order to exclude other diseases – possibly fueled by fears of malpractice litigation. Such investigations are often unnecessary, expensive and expose the child to radiation or other trauma. In the child with recurrent episodes of wheezing it is likely that some investigations will have already been undertaken in a previous attack and these should not be repeated unless there are very clear indications to do so. Acute RSV viral bronchiolitis and the investigations required in such patients or infants with moderate or severe wheezing for the first time is considered in Chapter 2.

Simple chest radiology

In the infant or preschool child with recurrent wheezing, and who has not had a previous chest radiograph, a plain postero–anterior and lateral films should be requested because it is impossible to be certain that there are no unusual features to the disease without them. For the infant with first time wheezing this is probably unnecessary, unless there are unusual features, but for the older infant or preschool child in whom foreign-body aspiration is always a possibility even first time wheezers should have a chest radiograph. No clinician is able to detect all serious intrathoracic abnormalities purely by physical examination. If recent films are available either they should be inspected or the opinion of a competent pediatric radiologist should be sought; new films should not be taken unless there are any unusual features. It should be remembered that some adult radiologists unfamiliar with pediatric chest films tend to report abnormalities which are of no real significance. In the large majority of typical wheezy infants the chest radiograph is normal or shows symmetrical bilateral hyperinflation. Minor areas of atelectasis may sometimes be found, especially in the middle lobe, but other infiltrates or abnormalities should not be present and would indicate the need for further investigation.

Computerized tomography (CT) scanning and other radiological studies

Unless there are very good reasons, CT scans are not indicated in the typical wheezy infant or preschool child and merely expose the child to quite unnecessary radiation.

Oxygen saturation

Pulse oximeters are now widely available and provide simple estimates of arterial blood oxygenation provided they are used correctly. For a reliable measurement the child must not be moving the hand or foot where the sensor is placed and the device should be displaying a steady signal of saturation and, if available, of heart rate. An erratic or variable signal is an unreliable index of saturation. In most wheezy children saturation will be normal; if it is low, and measured reliably, it is an indication of severe obstruction or some other pulmonary problem.

BHR

BHR is a cardinal feature of asthma and may also occur in certain other types of chronic lung disease. Subjects with BHR develop airways obstruction, and hence wheeze, more readily than normal subjects in response to certain stimuli which may occur naturally, such as physical exercise or the hyperventilation associated with crying, or may be induced by the inhalation of agents such as methacholine or adenosine 5' monophosphate. Inhalation challenges can be performed in the very young child and have a place in differential diagnosis but are not necessary for the routine management of the typical wheezy infant or preschool child.

Allergy and other investigations

These investigations are rarely indicated for the diagnosis and management of the large majority of typical wheezy infants and preschool children. There is evidence that the presence of eosinophilia in the young wheezy child is predictive of the subsequent development of asthma.[33] An elevated level of total IgE has also been shown to be a marker for later asthma.[34] Skin tests for allergy are all but useless at this age and may well be negative to common allergens even in an atopic infant. A sweat test or DNA analysis for CF and immunologic investigations are not indicated in the typical wheezy infant. However, given the considerable variation in the CF phenotype, many pediatricians would feel it obligatory to obtain a sweat test in an infant with troublesome, recurrent wheezing. Tests of lung function can be undertaken in specialized centers in infants less than about 18 months of age. These are discussed more fully in Chapter 5.

MANAGEMENT DECISIONS

During an attack

After taking the history and examining the child a decision has to be made as to whether or not further investigations are needed and how to manage the patient. Except in severely ill infants, investigations, if indicated, can usually be undertaken electively. The essential decisions when the child is seen in the clinic are concerned with where the child should be treated and whether or not there is the need to start medication. Unless the child is very distressed when first seen, with signs equivalent to a score of approximately ≥ 10 according to the scoring system shown in Tables 4.1 and 4.2, it should be possible to manage the problem on an ambulatory basis in the normal home environment. However, if there are adverse home circumstances it may be preferable to treat the child in a hospital day-care facility until the condition is stabilized. If the child is more distressed, a decision has to be made as to whether or not to refer him/her directly to the hospital emergency department. If the child is too breathless to feed normally, if the child is centrally cyanosed or the oxygen saturation breathing air is below about 92–93%, referral to the emergency department is recommended. The reason is that the child may well require inspired oxygen and intravenous fluids, and there is always the small but real possibility of respiratory arrest. Similar considerations apply when the infant is seen in the emergency department concerning the need for transfer to the pediatric intensive care unit. In this case, it is the possibility of the need for intubation and ventilation which usually determines whether or not the child stays in the emergency department, is admitted to the pediatric ward or is transferred to the intensive care unit. Oxygen saturation alone may not be an adequate indicator in this situation and arterial blood gas measurement is needed to determine whether pCO_2 is elevated and especially whether it is rising despite treatment.

The child with recurrent wheezing

The decision about medication for the typical infant or preschool child with recurrent wheezing is problematic. On the one hand, the large majority of such infants neither need nor respond to medications. On the other hand, parents are often very justifiably concerned and expect the doctor to do something that will help. If the child is not unduly distressed, is able to feed normally and is not hypoxic, either clinically or when measured by pulse oximetry, it may be possible to explain the nature of the problem to the parents and adopt a wait-and-see policy before trying medication. If the child is more distressed or if the parents are anxious because of the frequency or perceived severity of the attacks it is almost impossible to avoid trying medication. There can be no hard and fast rules here and the tolerance of parents (and their doctors) for symptoms in the wheezy child varies widely. If the decision is made to try medication then the rule should be that the simpler and safer the regimen the better. Most would recommend trying the effect of a simple short acting β_2-agonist bronchodilator on an as-needed basis delivered by a jet-type nebulizer to an open face mask. The use of other medications is discussed in Chapter 7 but whatever treatment is prescribed it is essential to be sure that it is of real value by careful clinical observation, especially when using medications with potential harmful effects such as corticosteroids.

What to tell the parents of the typical wheezy infant or preschool child

Every parent of a wheezy infant or preschool child wants to know whether their child has asthma, whether on not the child will grow out of it and does the child need long-term treatment. The epidemiology of the wheezy infant and preschool child is considered more fully in Chapter 1 but certain aspects inevitably impinge on management decisions.

Does the wheezy infant or preschool child really have asthma?

Some of these children will be true asthmatics who have inherited those genes which have enabled them to develop the type of allergic airway inflammation leading to BHR. These children are likely to have all or most of the following features:

- a personal or family history of asthma or allergies including infantile eczema;
- discrete attacks with completely symptom-free intervals;
- symptoms worse at night;
- apparent good response to bronchodilators or corticosteroids if used;
- normal plain chest radiograph or just hyperinflation;
- eosinophilia and elevated total IgE;
- positive bronchial provocation challenge (PCwheeze – see Chapter 5).

A clinical scoring system was developed by Castro-Rodriguez and co-workers[35] which was based on the frequency of early wheezing, wheezing without obvious colds, physician-diagnosed asthma, eczema and rhinitis, and eosinophilia (Box 4.1). Using this scoring system, 59% of infants with a positive loose index and 76% of those with a positive stringent index developed asthma during follow-up. However, there are infants and preschool children who have a very similar clinical pattern of illness but without the atopic background (the non-atopic wheezers) and in whom wheezing attacks are principally due to recurrent viral infections. Currently, there appear to be no good methods of distinguishing these young viral-induced wheezers from the young asthmatics apart from the atopic background, and even this may be unreliable since the asthma may appear before the atopic features.

Will the child grow out of the wheezing illness?

To complicate matters, it is far from clear what the relationship is between asthma and viral-related wheezing in young children. In a recent study by Sigurs et al[36] there was a significant increase in asthma at 7.5 years of age in children who had suffered from RSV

Box 4.1 The clinical index to define the risk of asthma in young children (taken from the data of Castro-Rodriguez et al[33])

Stringent Index
Early frequent wheezing (≥ 3 on a scale of 0–5) during first three years of life

Loose Index
Early wheezing (1–2 on a scale of 0–5) in the first three years of life

Both indices with:
   either medically diagnosed asthma (by history) or medically diagnosed atopic dermatitis
   (by parental questionnaire) or two out of three of medically diagnosed allergic rhinitis
   (by parental questionnaire)
   wheezing without colds
   eosinophilia ≥ 4%

---

bronchiolitis in infancy. In this study the cumulative prevalence of asthma was 30% in the RSV group and 3% in the control group ($P < 0.001$), and the cumulative prevalence of any wheezing was 68 and 34%, respectively ($P < 0.001$). Asthma during the year prior to follow-up was seen in 23% of the RSV children and 2% in the control subjects ($P < 0.001$). Allergic sensitization was found in 41% of the RSV children and 22% of the control subjects ($P = 0.039$). However, it is noteworthy that only four of the 47 (15%) asthmatics at 7.5 years of age from the RSV group were atopic and therefore 85% were non-atopic. These children could have come from the group we have defined as non-atopic wheezy infants in whom BHR had been induced by the original RSV infection.

Other follow-up studies have shown that infants with RSV bronchiolitis have a disease of limited duration and do not suffer from classical childhood asthma later. Some years ago, Pullan and Hey[7] undertook a long-term controlled study of infants with proven RSV bronchiolitis and found that 38% of the RSV group of infants had repeated episodes of mild wheezing compared with 15% of the controls over the first four years of life. By 10 years of age only 6.2% of the RSV group and 4.5% of the control group were wheezing. In a prospective cohort study, Martinez et al[2] found that approximately 40% of infants who wheezed for the first time before 3 years of age never wheezed again up to the second evaluation at 6 years of age. There was some evidence to suggest that the children who wheezed before 3 years of age and then stopped wheezing were different from those who continued to wheeze (Table 4.3). Very similar conclusions can be drawn from other studies which have shown that there are differences in the prognosis of infants who wheezed due to viral infections compared with those who began to wheeze later or had an atopic personal or family background.[37] A meta-analysis looking at this problem was undertaken by Kneyber et al,[8] who found six studies which met their selection criteria adequately. Up to 5 years of follow-up after RSV bronchiolitis in infancy, 40% of children reported wheezing as compared to only 11% in the control group ($P < 0.001$). Between 5 and 10 years of follow-up, 22% of the bronchiolitis group reported wheezing compared to 10% of the control group ($P = 0.19$). The incidence of recurrent wheezing as defined by three or more wheezing episodes also decreased with increasing years of follow-up: at 5 or more years of follow-up the difference between the

Table 4.3 Factors associated with different patterns of wheezing in infants and young children (from the data of Martinez et al[2])

	Wheezed only < 3 years of age	Wheezed < 3 years of age and continued
V'maxFRC < 1 year of age*	Reduced	Normal
Mother smokes	Yes	No
Mother with asthma	No	Yes
IgE	Normal	Elevated
Skin tests	Negative	Positive

* Forced expiratory flow at resting lung volume.

RSV group and the control group was no longer significant. Furthermore, the presence of either a personal and/or a family history of either atopy and/or asthma did not differ between the two groups. They concluded that, 'It seems unlikely that RSV bronchiolitis is a cause of atopic asthma in later life.'

Putting all this in perspective and in simple terms it can be concluded that:

- most wheezy infants < 1 year of age who have had more than one episode of wheezing are likely to have more episodes over the next few months or even for 3–4 years;
- if the infant has no personal or family background of allergy and especially if the illness began during the winter RSV season, the chances of the disease being limited to infancy are great and the likelihood of later childhood asthma are small;
- if the infant has a personal or family history of allergy and especially if the illness began outside the RSV season, the likelihood that this is asthma is greater and the disease may well continue into later childhood.

Since it can be estimated that roughly 20% of all children are potential asthmatics and carry the asthma genes, then by chance 20% of those who suffer from RSV (or other viral) bronchiolitis are also potential asthmatics and the virus may induce them to become true asthmatics. At present there are no tests which distinguish with certainty which wheezy infant < 1 year of age is the atopic and which is the non-atopic wheezer.

Does the child need long-term treatment?

In older infants and preschool children non-atopic wheezing may be due to repeated viral infections but it is currently impossible to distinguish these children from true asthmatics. Because it is often impossible to know whether the recurrent wheezy child is asthmatic or has viral-related wheezing, the approach to treatment is usually the same for all of them. This includes:

- commencement of therapy using appropriate inhalation techniques (see Chapter 7);
- avoidance of unnecessary administration of antibiotics;

- careful follow up to ensure that:
  treatment is being given correctly
  the symptoms are well controlled
  no need for more treatment
  no need for less treatment
  no adverse effects
  the child does indeed have atopic or non-atopic wheezing and other diagnoses have been excluded.

In this way we can try to determine the need for long-term treatment. For those who respond to treatment, parents wish to know when the child can stop medication and this is usually a question of trial and error. As to the question whether or not treatment can 'cure' the condition or hasten its spontaneous resolution, to be perfectly honest, there are presently no certain answers and more research is needed.

CLINICAL FEATURES OF THE ATYPICAL WHEEZY INFANT AND PRESCHOOL CHILD

While by far the most of common causes of wheezing in this age group are atopic and non-atopic wheezing, there are a number of other very important conditions in which the clinical picture is similar but which, if misdiagnosed, can result in very serious and even fatal consequences for the child. Careful attention to the clinical features may provide clues suggesting that the problem is not typical and these are briefly reviewed here and more fully, along with the differential diagnosis, in Chapter 6. It is important to remember that in countries where tuberculosis is common, this may be present in addition to atopic or non-atopic wheezing and this possibility should always be kept in mind when evaluating the child. A summary of important differences between typical and atypical wheezing is given in Table 4.4.

Atypical features from the history

There are a number of features in the history which should alert the physician to the possibility that the problem is not necessarily the usual type of wheezy infant or preschool child. These include:

- symptoms dating from birth or shortly afterwards;
- wheeze which is continuous throughout the 24 hours;
- wheeze which does not have definite attacks lasting a few days separated by clear symptom-free (or largely symptom-free) intervals of weeks or months;
- failure to thrive;
- total failure to respond to anti-asthmatic medications is suggestive, but many young children with typical causes of wheeze also fail to respond.

Atypical features from physical examination

Important clues indicating a possible atypical cause of wheezing may be obtained by careful physical examination. These include:

- failure to thrive;

- asymmetry of the chest or bony anomalies such as pectus excavatum;[38]
- unilateral or localized wheezing or reduced air entry;
- monophonic wheeze, especially that which is purely inspiratory;
- crackles, marked tachypnea and central cyanosis other than during a severe exacerbation;
- clubbing of the nails;
- marked upper respiratory tract or ear disease are often associated with other causes of wheezing;
- neurologic impairment which may be a cause of aspiration.

Investigations in suspected atypical wheezing

In the infant or preschool child with atypical wheezing according to the history or examination, certain investigations such as a plain chest radiograph are mandatory as physical examination alone is not accurate enough. In many situations only simple investigations are needed but the pediatrician must be aware when more complicated procedures are indicated. These include a CT scan of the chest, bronchoscopy, a

Table 4.4 Summary of features of typical and atypical wheezing in infancy and early childhood

	Typical wheeze	Atypical wheeze
History	Early onset more common	Any age
	Episodic attacks	More usually continuous
	Symptom-free intervals	Symptom-free intervals less common
	Possible personal atopy	Unrelated to atopy
	Possible family atopy	Unrelated to family atopy
	Possible viral infection	Unrelated to infection
	Unrelated to feeding	Possibly related to feeding
Examination	Normal development	May have failure to thrive
	No chest deformity	May have chest deformity
	No clubbing of the nails	May have clubbing of the nails
	No marked URT* disease	Possible severe URT* disease
	Generalized wheezing	May have localized wheezing
	Generalized reduced breath sounds	May have localized reduced breath sounds
	Musical polyphonic wheeze	May have coarse or monophonic wheeze
Investigations	Normal chest X-ray or generalized hyperinflation	May have localized hyperinflation on chest X-ray
	No infiltrates on chest X-ray, or only local changes	May have extensive infiltrates on chest X-ray
	Possible elevated IgE	Unrelated to IgE
	Possible eosinophilia	Unrelated to eosinophilia

* Upper respiratory tract.

barium swallow and studies of the upper gastrointestinal tract or overnight monitoring of esophageal pH to look for evidence of reflux and aspiration. Echocardiography is indicated to seek evidence of a vascular ring or unsuspected congenital heart disease compressing the airway. Other special investigations will depend upon the clinical picture and the tests most likely to provide useful information. Bronchoscopy now plays a major role in the diagnosis of congenital and acquired disorders in infants and young children, and the yield from this procedure is very high provided the patients are properly selected.[39] Besides the diagnosis and removal of foreign bodies from the airways, bronchoscopy is the most efficient method of diagnosing many congenital airway anomalies, and obtaining evidence of aspiration and infection. The indications and uses of plain radiology, contrast radiology, CT scans, lung function tests and bronchoscopy in the atypical wheezy infant or preschool child are discussed more fully in Chapter 6.

Management decisions and prognosis in atypical wheezing

The essential management decision that the general pediatrician should make is that further investigation is required for an infant or preschool child whose wheezing is atypical. Unless the child is seriously ill or foreign-body aspiration is suspected, most investigations can be undertaken electively. Apart from arranging for a plain chest radiograph and perhaps a sweat test or other simple basic investigations, most decisions concerning CT scans, bronchoscopy or other more invasive procedures should usually be undertaken in consultation with a specialist in pediatric pulmonology. The prognosis in the atypical wheezy infant or preschool child obviously depends upon the nature of the problem. It may be necessary to spend some time explaining the possibilities to the parents who may well feel that their wheezy child is just the same as their other wheezy children or those of friends.

REFERENCES

1. Smith DH, Malone DC, Lawson KA et al. A national estimate of the economic costs of asthma. *Am J Respir Crit Care Med* 1997; **156**: 787–93.

2. Martinez FD, Wright AL, Taussig LM et al and the Group Health Medical Associates. Asthma and wheezing in the first six years of life. *N Engl J Med* 1995; **332**: 133–8.

3. Young S, Arnott J, O'Keeffe PT et al. The association between early life lung function and wheezing during the first 2 yrs of life. *Eur Respir J* 2000; **15**: 151–7.

4. Kuehni CE, Davis A, Brooke AM, Silverman M. Are all wheezing disorders in very young (preschool) children increasing in prevalence? *Lancet* 2001; **357**: 1821–5.

5. Rusconi F, Galassi C, Corbo GM et al. Risk factors for early, persistent, and late-onset wheezing in young children. SIDRIA Collaborative Group. *Am J Respir Crit Care Med* 1999; **160**: 1617–22.

6. Oddy WH, De Kock MA, Sly PD, Holt PG. The effects of respiratory infections, atopy, and breastfeeding on childhood asthma. *Eur Respir J* 2002; **19**: 899–905.

7. Pullan CR, Hey EN. Wheezing, asthma and pulmonary dysfunction 10 years after infection with respiratory syncytial

virus in infancy. *Br Med J* 1982; **284**: 1665–9.

8. Kneyber MCJ, Steyerberg EW, de Groot R, Moll HA. Long-term effects of respiratory syncytial virus (RSV) bronchiolitis in infants and young children: a quantitative review. *Acta Paediatr* 2000; **89**: 654–60.

9. Reijonen TM, Kotaniemi-Syrjanen A, Korhonen K, Korppi M. Predictors of asthma three years after hospital admission for wheezing in infancy. *Pediatrics* 2000; **106**: 1406–12.

10. Young S, Arnott J, Le Souef PN, Landau LI. Flow limitation during tidal expiration in symptom-free infants and the subsequent development of asthma. *J Pediatr* 1994; **124**: 681–8.

11. Martinez FD, Morgan WJ, Wright AL et al and the Group Health Medical Associates' Personnel. Diminished lung function as a predisposing factor for wheezing respiratory illness in infants. *N Engl J Med* 1988; **319**: 1112–17.

12. The International Study of Asthma and Allergies in Childhood (ISAAC). Worldwide variation in prevalence of symptoms of asthma, allergic rhinoconjunctivitis, and atopic eczema: ISAAC. *Lancet* 1998; **351**: 1225–32.

13. Dawson B, Horrobin G, Illesley R, Mitchell R. A survey of childhood asthma in Aberdeen. *Lancet* 1969; **1**: 827–30.

14. Aberg N, Engstrom I. Natural history of allergic diseases in childhood. *Acta Paediatr Scand* 1990; **79**: 206–11.

15. Ponsonby AL, Gatenby P, Glasgow N et al. Which clinical subgroups within the spectrum of child asthma are attributable to atopy? *Chest* 2002; **121**: 135–42.

16. National Institute of Health (NIH). *Global strategy for asthma management and prevention*. (NIH: Bethesda, MD, 2002.)

17. Einarsson O, Geba GP, Zhu Z et al. Interleukin-11: stimulation in vivo and in vitro by respiratory viruses and induction of airways hyperresponsiveness. *J Clin Invest* 1996; **97**: 915–24.

18. Mckean MC, Leech M, Lambert PC et al. A model of viral wheeze in nonasthmatic adults: symptoms and physiology. *Eur Respir J* 2001; **18**: 23–32.

19. Welliver RC, Duffy L. The relationship of RSV-specific immunoglobulin E antibody response in infancy, recurrent wheezing, and pulmonary function at age 7–8 years. *Pediatr Pulmonol* 1993; **15**: 19–27.

20. Cane RS, Ranganathan SC, McKenzie SA. What do parents of wheezy children understand by 'wheeze'? *Arch Dis Child* 2000; **82**: 327–32.

21. Cane RS, McKenzie SA. Parents' interpretations of children's respiratory symptoms on video. *Arch Dis Child* 2001; **84**: 31–4.

22. Lee H, Arroyo A, Rosenfeld W. Parents' evaluations of wheezing in their children with asthma. *Chest* 1996; **109**: 91–3.

23. Cserhati E, Mezei G, Kelemen J. Late prognosis of bronchial asthma in children. *Respiration* 1984; **46**: 160–5.

24. Godfrey S, Bar-Yishay E. Exercise-induced asthma revisited. *Respir Med* 1993; **87**: 331–44.

25. Tariq SM, Matthews SM, Hakim EA et al. The prevalence of and risk factors for atopy in early childhood: a whole population birth cohort study. *J Allergy Clin Immunol* 1998; **101**: 587–93.

26. de Jong MH, Scharp-van der Linden VTM, Aalberse RC et al. Randomised controlled trial of a brief neonatal exposure to cow's milk on the development of atopy. *Arch Dis Child* 1998; **79**: 126–30.

27. Hill DJ, Duke AM, Hosking CS, Hudson IL. Clinical manifestations of cows' milk allergy in childhood. II. The diagnostic value of skin tests and RAST. *Clin Allergy* 1988; **18**: 481–90.

28. Tager IB, Hanrahan JP, Tosteson TD et al. Lung function, pre- and post-natal smoke exposure, and wheezing in the first year of life. *Am Rev Respir Dis* 1993; **147**: 811–17.

29. Wilson AC, Forsyth JS, Greene SA et al. Relation of infant diet to childhood health: seven year follow up of cohort of children in Dundee infant feeding study. *Br Med J* 1998; **316**: 21–5.

30. Gavriely N, Palti Y, Alroy G, Grotberg JB. Measurement and theory of wheezing

breath sounds. *J Appl Physiol* 1988; **57**: 481–92.

31. Tal A, Bavilski C, Yohai D et al. Dexamethasone and salbutamol in the treatment of acute wheezing in infants. *Pediatrics* 1983; **71**: 13–18.

32. Bertrand P, Aranibar H, Castro E, Sanchez I. Efficacy of nebulized epinephrine versus salbutamol in hospitalized infants with bronchiolitis. *Pediatr Pulmonol* 2001; **31**: 284–8.

33. Castro-Rodriguez JA, Holberg CJ, Wright AL, Martinez F. A clinical index to define risk of asthma in young children with recurrent wheezing. *Am J Respir Crit Care Med* 2000; **162**: 1403–6.

34. Klinnert MD, Nelson HS, Price MR et al. Onset and persistence of childhood asthma: predictors from infancy. *Pediatrics* 2001; **108**: E69.

35. Ball TM, Castro-Rodriguez JA, Griffith KA et al. Siblings, day-care attendance, and the risk of asthma and wheezing during childhood. *N Engl J Med* 2000; **343**: 538–43.

36. Sigurs N, Bjarnason R, Sigurbergsson F, Kjellman B. Respiratory syncytial virus bronchiolitis in infancy is an important risk factor for asthma and allergy at age 7. *Am J Respir Crit Care Med* 2000; **161**: 1501–7.

37. Sporik R, Holgate ST, Cogswell JJ. Natural history of asthma in childhood – a birth cohort study. *Arch Dis Child* 1991; **66**: 1050–3.

38. Godfrey S. Association between pectus excavatum and segmental bronchomalacia. *J Pediatr* 1980; **96**: 649–52.

39. Godfrey S, Avital A, Maayan C et al. Yield from flexible bronchoscopy in children. *Pediatr Pulmonol* 1997; **23**: 261–9.

5
Lung function in the wheezy infant and preschool child

BASIC PULMONARY PHYSIOLOGY RELEVANT TO DISORDERS ASSOCIATED WITH WHEEZING

The functions of the lungs include the mechanics of moving gas to and from the gas-exchanging regions through the non-exchanging dead space of the tracheobronchial tree and the exchange of gases between the alveoli and pulmonary capillary blood. The main functional disturbance in infants and young children who wheeze, as in older children and adults, is obstruction principally of the smaller airways. In most disorders associated with wheezing, disturbance to the mechanical function of the lungs results in varying degrees of mismatching of alveolar ventilation and perfusion. This in turn disturbs gas exchange, chiefly of oxygen, and causes some degree of hypoxemia.

Movement of gas from the atmosphere to and from the alveoli depends upon the mechanical properties of the lungs and thorax that form the pump, and the respiratory muscles which contribute the driving force. In disorders associated with wheezing there is no reason why there should be any problem with the respiratory muscles although, if the thorax becomes very hyperinflated, the muscles may have to work at a mechanical disadvantage. The performance of the respiratory pump, like any other bellows-type pump, depends upon the size (volume) of the pump, the material of which it is constructed, which affects the force needed to change its shape, and, most importantly, the resistance of the conducting airway through which the gas must flow. The properties of the materials of which the respiratory pump are constructed, namely the lung tissue and thorax, are usually normal in lung diseases associated with wheezing. However, there is one important exception: in wheezy infants with congenital heart disease causing increased pulmonary blood flow, the lung tissue is abnormally stiff and the lung compliance (volume change per unit of applied pressure) is reduced. While the primary functional disturbance in diseases associated with wheezing is related to the resistance to gas flow through the conducting airways, lung volume may be secondarily affected by the trapping of gas during expiration, resulting in a greater than normal end expiratory lung volume, the functional residual capacity (FRC).

The resistance (pressure gradient needed to produce unit gas flow) of the conducting airways is the central factor in determining lung function in disorders associated with wheezing. These airways form a branching system that is more or less dichotomous from the trachea (termed generation 0) to the main bronchi (generation 1) and on down through many generations to the respiratory bronchioles. At each division, the effective cross-section of the airway is increased because the sum of the cross-sections of the daughter bronchi is greater than that of the parent. The smallest cross-sectional area in the bronchial tree is at the level of the vocal cords. The increasing cross-sectional area distal to the trachea reduces the resistance to gas flow as the airways get smaller. Even though the diameter of the small airways (about < 1–2 mm in diameter) are much less than the more proximal large airways, the huge number of parallel pathways, their greatly increased combined cross-sectional area and their shorter length means that these very critical small airways contribute very little to the total airways resistance in health (and even in disease).

This is not to say that the small airways are without any effect on gas flow, especially during forced or maximal expiration. When lung volume decreases during expiration in subjects in whom the resistance of the small airways is increased by disease, there is sufficient pressure drop between the alveoli and the larger airways to cause collapse of these relatively flaccid larger airways in such a way that no matter how much force is applied, the pressure drop across this segment of the airway remains constant. Since flow is equal to pressure divided by resistance, and the resistance of the diseased small airways is relatively constant in a given disease state and the driving pressure is also constant, maximal expiratory flow is constant and reduced below normal irrespective of the effort used by the subject. This explanation of the phenomenon is based on what is termed the equal pressure point theory but it is equally well explained by the wave speed theory of the propagation of gases in a tube, which predicts that maximum expiratory flow is limited by the properties of the airways and independent of effort. The theoretical details are unimportant in clinical practice but the effect is very important indeed, since this explains why maximal expiratory flow at low lung volume is limited in obstructive lung disease due primarily to disease of the small airways. It is also the basis of possibly the most important of all measures of lung function at all ages, including infancy, i.e. the parameters derived from the forced expiratory flow–volume (F–V) loop.

In obstructive lung diseases there is increased resistance to airflow, chiefly during expiration, when lung volume and airway caliber become smaller, and this obstruction may either be fixed, as in diseases such as bronchiolitis obliterans, or variable, such as in asthma. The wide fluctuations in airway resistance spontaneously or in response to treatment [bronchial hyperresponsiveness (BHR)] are a cardinal feature of asthma, and measurement of this property of the airways is important theoretically and clinically. In asthma, the reversible airway obstruction is due both to bronchospasm, which is largely reversed by a bronchodilator, or to more subtle airway inflammation, which may be reversed by corticosteroids. The degree of bronchial responsiveness may be evaluated by repeated measurements of lung function but more usually either by measuring the effect of a bronchodilator or corticosteroid on lung function, or by deliberately attempting to provoke bronchoconstriction by exposure to some type of chemical or physical stimulus.

HOW ARE TESTS OF LUNG FUNCTION USED CLINICALLY IN OLDER SUBJECTS WITH OBSTRUCTIVE LUNG DISEASES?

In older subjects with wheezing disorders, the diagnosis, evaluation of severity and response to treatment is substantially improved by the use of appropriate tests of lung function. Techniques are available for the measurement of total airway resistance, which mainly reflects the function of the larger airways, and indirect techniques exist which reflect the resistance of the smaller airways. Lung volume and its subdivisions can also be measured, which is helpful in some situations because airway caliber is dependent upon lung volume. The simplest and most useful clinical parameters of lung function in older patients are derived from forced expiratory F–V loops or simple spirometry (which in reality is just an alternative way of expressing the same relationships). While it is possible to measure pulmonary compliance in older subjects, this is a difficult and complicated procedure and is chiefly used for research purposes. Disturbances of ventilation–perfusion matching are reflected in arterial hypoxemia and, for most purposes, this can now be determined non-invasively by pulse oximetry.

For many subjects with wheezing disorders it is not enough to measure lung function under baseline resting conditions since this may not reflect the true nature of the functional disturbance. The asthmatic may have normal or virtually normal lung function between attacks. Even when there is an obstructive defect in lung function at rest this must be distinguished from the findings in other types of chronic obstructive pulmonary disease (COPD), chiefly by the demonstration of reversibility or BHR. Bronchial responsiveness is measured by exposing the subject to an appropriate stimulus, which acts either directly on the bronchial smooth muscle (agents such as inhaled histamine or methacholine) or through intermediate metabolic pathways [physical exercise, inhaled allergen or inhaled adenosine 5′-monophosphate (AMP)]. The response in older children and adults to the challenge is evaluated by the measurement of lung function, usually by spirometry.

In older children and adults with wheezing disorders, tests of lung function are used to answer a number of important clinical questions:

- is there any evidence of reduced lung function at the time of testing?
- if lung function is abnormal, is the abnormality of the obstructive type such as found in asthma, cystic fibrosis (CF) and other types of COPD?
- to what extent is the abnormal lung function reversible in the short term by the inhalation of a bronchodilator agent?
- to what extent is the abnormal lung function reversible in the long term by the administration of a corticosteroid or other medication?;
- does the patient demonstrate an abnormal degree of bronchial responsiveness on exposure to appropriate stimuli?
- to what extent does lung function vary over weeks or months, either spontaneously or in response to treatment?

Based on the answers to these questions, along with other clinical data, decisions are reached as to the diagnosis and correct treatment for the patient.

LUNG FUNCTION TESTS FOR THE VERY YOUNG

Difficulties in performing tests

The situation with the infant and preschool child is essentially no different from that in older patients, but the measurement of lung function in these young patients is much more difficult, time consuming, costly and, sometimes, impossible. Problems in the measurement of lung function in the very young patient include the following.

- Infants and young children are unable to cooperate actively with the tests, and most are unwilling to tolerate face masks, mouthpieces or other items of respiratory equipment, and have a natural fear of all medical procedures.
- Sedation is needed in all but the newborn infant in order to get the child to tolerate a face mask and other respiratory equipment. In children between about 2 and 4–5 years of age the measurement of the mechanical functions of the lung is virtually impossible on a routine basis without deep sedation or anesthesia, which is rarely, if ever, justified.
- The severity of the illness may render it unsafe to undertake measurements of lung function even under light sedation.
- Parents (and some physicians) are nervous about submitting infants to tests of lung function, especially when they can see no immediate benefit from the procedure.
- There is a lack of standardized, commercially available equipment for the measurement of lung function in infants and young children.
- There is a relative lack of information on lung function in normal infants and young children.

Techniques that are suitable

It is now over half a century since the late Kenneth Cross and his colleagues began to make objective measurements of ventilation and the control of breathing in newborn infants,[1,2] and over 40 years since investigators made the first reliable measurements of the mechanical function of the lungs in healthy and sick infants.[3–5] These early studies were mostly made using a head out plethysmograph to measure tidal volume combined with an esophageal balloon to measure pleural pressure, which allowed pulmonary resistance and compliance to be calculated. Since then great strides have been made both in the development of equipment and the way in which tests are performed. The modern approach to lung function testing in infancy has recently been summarized by investigators from the American Thoracic and European Respiratory societies.[6]

Without any doubt, the simplest and most practical test of lung function in the first 12–18 months of life is the measurement of forced expiratory flow from a partial or complete forced expiratory F–V loop. Another relatively simple technique is to measure face mask pressure, reflecting alveolar pressure, and flow during induced passive expiration from elevated lung volume, which provides information on the resistance and compliance of the total respiratory system, provided the resistance of the smaller airways is not markedly increased. The whole-body infant plethysmograph is much more complicated to use but with modern computer techniques provides important information on lung volume and the changes of resistance during respiration. Airway resistance can also be estimated using forced oscillation applied at the mouth, and this is also relatively simple for the child provided that a good seal can be obtained with a face mask. None of these tests, possibly with the exception of forced oscillation measurements, are suitable for the routine investigation of older infants and preschool children because of the problem of cooperation. On the other hand, measurements of bronchial responsivity to inhaled agents can be undertaken in most older infants and preschool children using surrogates for the measurement of lung function, such as chest auscultation, to detect wheeze.

Forced expiration (V′max,FRC; FEV$_{0.5}$)

The first measurements of forced expiratory flow in infants were undertaken by Motoyama et al[7] using forced deflation of the lungs by the application of a negative pressure to anesthetized infants through an endotracheal tube. Later investigators made this much simpler by applying sudden compression of the thorax from an inflatable jacket at end inspiration while flow was measured at the mouth.[8–10] The equipment is simple, thoracic compression jackets can be purchased or made and the skill required to perform the test is easily acquired. Since these curves were obtained by squeezing at the end of a normal inspiration and not at the end of a maximal inspiration they were termed partial F–V curves. The characteristic shapes of a partial F–V curve from a normal infant and an acutely wheezy infant are shown in Figure 5.1. The convex shaped curve of the wheezy infant with respect to the volume axis is similar to the shape of an F–V curve in an older child or adult with obstructive lung disease. The most usual parameter derived from such an F–V curve is the maximum expiratory flow at FRC (resting lung volume), which is usually termed V′max,FRC. More recently, different methods have been used to obtain complete F–V curves in infants. These involve inducing apnea by a brief period of manual hyperventilation, inflating the lungs manually or automatically to a predetermined pressure (20–30 cm.H$_2$O) sufficient to increase lung volume to total lung capacity (TLC), and then applying the

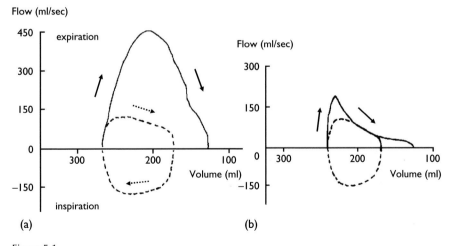

Figure 5.1

Partial expiratory flow–volume (F–V) curves from (a) a normal infant and (b) an acutely wheezy infant. In these infants lung volume was measured in the whole-body plethysmograph so that the volume axis shows absolute lung volume. The dashed lines show the tidal F–V loop preceding the forced expiration.

squeeze.[11,12] With this technique, lung volume is more standardized and it is also possible to derived time-based parameters, such as the forced expiratory volume (FEV) in the first 0.5 seconds ($FEV_{0.5}$), akin to parameters obtained from spirometry in older children. The technique is a little more complicated and it has yet to be shown convincingly that the information obtained is of greater clinical value than that obtained from a partial F–V curve. Useful information can be obtained by repeating the test after treatment and in some infants an excellent response may be observed (Figure 5.2), very like that in an older patient with asthma. Some investigators use the shape of the F–V curve obtained during tidal breathing rather than forced expiration to derive parameters reflecting the site and severity of airways obstruction, but there is less agreement on the value of this type of test as compared with tests of forced expiration.

Passive expiration respiratory system compliance (C_{rs}) and resistance (R_{rs})

The respiratory system can be modeled by assuming that it resembles a simple electrical circuit containing a resistance (R) and capacitance (C; compliance) in series. In such a system, when the circuit is closed, the current discharges at a rate dependent upon R and C such that a plot of the current (flow) versus voltage (volume) is a straight line, the slope of which is the time constant (τ) of the system. The relationships between flow and pressure in the lungs for this purpose can only be determined when the respiratory muscles are relaxed. This is obtained by briefly occluding the airway during expiration to inhibit the respiratory muscles through the Hering–Breuer reflex. When the

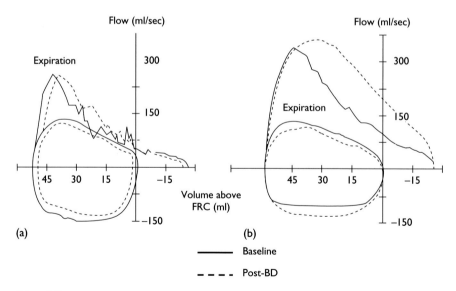

Figure 5.2

Forced expired flow–volume (F–V) loops from an infant of 9 months of age showing (a) no response initially in the obstructive pattern to an inhaled bronchodilator (BD) and (b) a marked improvement in both baseline lung function and bronchodilator responsiveness after 1 month of treatment with an oral corticosteroid on an alternate-day basis. (FRC, functional residual capacity.)

occlusion is released, the decline of expiratory flow plotted versus the decreasing lung volume (Figure 5.3a) gives the time constant of the respiratory system (τ_{rs}). Extrapolation of the line to zero flow gives the total relaxed volume that could have been exhaled and, knowing the mouth pressure at the time of the relaxed occlusion, the respiratory system compliance can be calculated (C_{rs} = volume/pressure). Respiratory system resistance (R_{rs} = flow/pressure) can be derived by analogy with the electrical circuit where $R_{rs} = \tau_{rs}/C_{rs}$.[13,14] This technique is simple to apply to young infants but suffers from one major drawback. The theory assumes that the lung can be considered as a single compartment model, which is reasonable for infants with normal lungs but inappropriate for infants with obstructive lung disease in whom there are many compartments with differing resistances and compliances. In such a multicompartment model, the plot of expiratory flow versus volume is not linear but convex to the volume axis (Figure 5.3b), and there is no single value for its slope and, hence, no single value for R or C.[15] This makes this technique of very dubious value in the wheezy infant.

Multiple occlusion respiratory system compliance (C_{rs})

Another technique based on passive expiration to measure C_{rs} was originally described for use in infants by Olinsky et al.[16] In this method, occlusions of the airway are made at different portions of the respiratory cycle and the volume above resting lung volume and the mouth pressure during occlusion are measured. Originally, occlusions were made during inspiration but now it is usual to make them during expiration. Assuming that the Hering–Breuer reflex relaxes the respiratory muscles, the mouth pressure at the time of occlusion can be related to the volume in the lungs above the fully relaxed

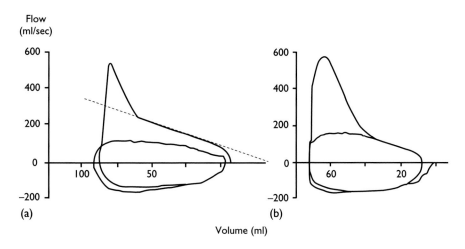

Figure 5.3

(a) Decline of expiratory flow versus the decreasing lung volume during passive expiration in an infant without small airways obstruction. The time constant of the respiratory system (τ_{rs}) is calculated from the linear portion of the expiration. (b) Similar plot from a wheezy infant in whom there is no clearly defined linear portion of the expiratory slope. In these infants absolute lung volume was not measured and the volume axis shows the volume above end expiratory lung volume from the preceding breath.

end expiratory volume. By plotting the volume versus pressure for the multiple points a graph can be drawn the slope of which is C_{rs} (Figure 5.4). This quasi-static measurement is largely independent of R_{rs} and so can be applied to almost all wheezy infants. This test can be very helpful in differential diagnosis, since wheezy infants with increased pulmonary blood flow due to cardiac disease have a low C_{rs}.

Forced oscillation (R_{rs})

This technique, which is of immediate appeal to the pediatric pulmonologist because it does not interfere with normal breathing, consists of applying a small sinusoidal oscillating pressure to the airway superimposed upon tidal breathing and measuring the

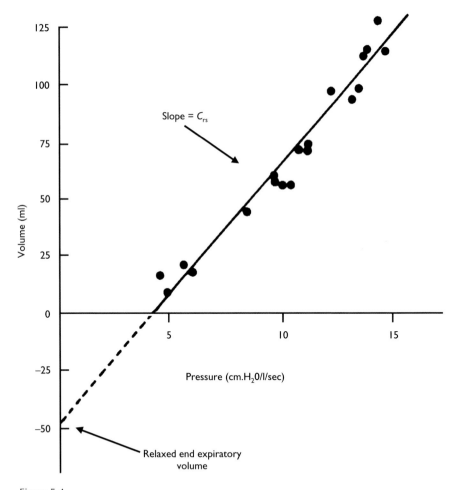

Figure 5.4

Multiple occlusion technique for measuring respiratory system compliance (C_{rs}). The slope of the regression of volume on pressure gives C_{rs}. In addition, the projection of the regression line to zero pressure shows the theoretical relaxed end expiratory volume, which is less than the actual end expiratory volume in this case.

induced changes in flow. The pressure can be applied through a face mask or alternatively by enclosing the head of the infant in a chamber to which the sinusoidal pressure is applied.[17] The technique is based on an analogy with the behavior of an electrical circuit to which a sinusoidal signal is applied and which contains a number of elements, the most relevant of which are resistance, capacitance and inertance. Using various computer models, the response of the respiratory system can be estimated in terms of resistance and compliance on the assumption that the lungs behave similarly to a simple electronic circuit. This technique has been used for many years in adults and in studies to evaluate the response of wheezy infants to the administration of a bronchodilator or bronchoconstrictor.[18–20] Unfortunately, the lungs of wheezy infants do not seem to behave as a simple electrical circuit and this results, among other things, in the estimate of resistance using forced oscillation, which depends on the applied frequency,[21] with no single value for resistance. Moreover, the values obtained for R_{rs} by forced oscillation often bear little relation to the values for airway resistance (R_{aw}) or parameters from forced expiration obtained by other methods,[22,23] which makes it difficult to know what exactly the forced oscillation technique is measuring. In a recent study by Hall et al,[20] forced oscillation was able to measure the bronchoconstrictor response to inhaled methacholine in only six out of 14 infants, while in all 14 there was a response as measured by the change in $FEV_{0.5}$ on forced expiration.

Infant whole-body plethysmography (R_{aw}, V_{tg})

The whole-body plethysmograph was originally developed by Dubois and his colleagues[24,25] for use in adults to measure lung volume and R_{aw}, and has been adopted with various modifications for use in infants and young children.[26–28] The plethysmograph consists of a closed chamber in which the infant lies and breathes through a respiratory circuit. By briefly obstructing the airway and simultaneously measuring the change in pressure on the lung side of the obstruction and that in the plethysmograph chamber, while the infant makes respiratory efforts against the occlusion, it is possible to calculate lung volume using Boyle's law. It is usual to calculate the volume remaining in the lungs at end expiration, which is termed the thoracic gas volume (V_{tg}). If the pressure changes in the plethysmograph chamber are related to the airflow at the mouth after the obstruction has been removed, but while the infant is breathing warmed and humidified air, it is possible to calculate R_{aw}. Because tissue resistance is very low in infants, R_{aw} is virtually identical to total respiratory resistance (R_{rs}). Using modern computer techniques, it is possible to measure resistance almost continuously throughout the respiratory cycle and thus to obtain the profile of the changing resistance during respiration.[28] The importance of such measurements is shown in Figure 5.5, where the difference between the rising inspiratory resistance due to upper airway obstruction is contrasted with the rising expiratory resistance due to small airways obstruction. This also emphasizes that resistance in infants with airways obstruction changes throughout the respiratory cycle and cannot be expressed by a single number, which explains why tests measuring R_{rs} based on passive expiration or forced oscillation are of limited value in wheezy infants. In some studies, V_{tg} in wheezy infants has been less than expected and this casts some doubt on the ability of plethysmography to measure lung mechanics

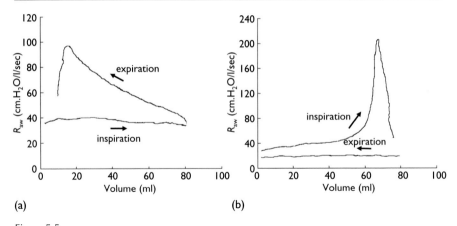

Figure 5.5

Airway resistance (R_{aw}) measured continuously throughout the respiratory cycle by whole-body plethysmography. (a) An infant with small airways obstruction in whom resistance rises towards the end of expiration. (b) An infant with laryngomalacia in whom the resistance rises towards the end of inspiration.

in such patients,[29] although it may well be that lungs and airways are indeed smaller in those infants prone to develop bronchiolitis.[30] Since R_{aw} is a measure of total airway resistance, of which only a relatively small part is due to the resistance of smaller airways, R_{aw} chiefly reflects large airway function. However, a prominent rise in R_{aw} towards late expiration indicates small airway disease because the small airways tend to close off as lung volume decreases and make a much greater contribution to R_{aw}. The major problem in the use of the whole-body plethysmograph to study lung function in infants is that the equipment and techniques are complicated, and the infant is required to sleep and breath regularly for some minutes through a face mask attached to the respiratory circuit. While some infants up to about 2 years of age can be studied in the plethysmograph, it is virtually impossible to study older infants.

Bronchial provocation in young children

Bronchial responsiveness is measured by administering increasing doses of the challenge agent by inhalation and recording the change in lung function. While it is possible to undertake inhalation bronchial challenges in infants using one of the techniques described above to measure lung function, the chances of completing the test are small because repeated measurement of lung function must be made as increasing doses of the challenge agent are administered. In many cases the infant wakes up before any response can be reliably detected. Children older than about 2–3 years of age with respiratory symptoms have often been treated with inhaled medications delivered to a loose-fitting face mask from a jet nebulizer. Such children will usually tolerate the administration of increasing doses of a challenge agent through a face mask while their response is evaluated by a surrogate for lung function such as the auscultation (PCwheeze) method or transcutaneous pO_2 ($ptcO_2$). There is now considerable experience with the auscultation method, which has proved to be simple and reliable.[31–33] In this technique, auscultation of the chest and pulse oximetry is used to determine the concentration of an agent such as methacholine (MCH) or AMP that provokes wheezing, tachypnea or mild desaturation. The inhalation is by a modification of the original tidal breathing method of Cockcroft et al,[34] in which fresh solutions of MCH or AMP are nebulized through a face mask during 2 minutes of tidal breathing, starting with a placebo solution and then followed by doubling concentrations of agent every 5 minutes until the maximal concentration or the end point is reached. Arterial oxygen saturation and heart rate are monitored continuously by pulse oximetry. The end point of a challenge is defined as wheezing heard with a stethoscope over the chest or the trachea, or a fall in oxygen saturation of at least 5% from baseline, or an increase in respiratory rate of at least 50% from baseline. Should oxygen saturation fall below 5% of baseline, nebulization of the agent is stopped immediately and a bronchodilator is given by nebulization driven by oxygen. In a study of 146 young children with asthma (mean of 4.3 years of age), Springer et al[33] found a positive response using the auscultation method in 95.9% of children (Table 5.1). Wheeze alone or in combination with other signs appeared in 81% of children. The mean desaturation at the end point was 4.6%, which compares with the 5.0% found in older children undergoing a conventional bronchial challenge. Sprikkelman et al[35] performed histamine challenges in older children with mild to moderate asthma and in 20 of 26 tests (77%) wheeze was present at the end point. Likewise, Yong et al[36] reported that methacholine challenges performed on 39 young children with a history of recurrent wheezing were terminated because of wheezing in 90% of tests. Other methods of performing bronchial challenges in young children include measurement of R_{rs} by forced oscillation and measurement of $ptcO_2$, but most agree that these techniques are less reliable.

Table 5.1 Signs appearing at the end point concentration of methacholine using the auscultation (PCwheeze) method in 146 young asthmatic preschool children (from Springer et al[33])

Signs at end point	No. of children (%)
With wheeze at end point	118 (80.8)
Wheeze alone	10 (6.8)
Wheeze + tachypnea	19 (13.0)
Wheeze + desaturation	20 (13.6)
Wheeze + tachypnea + desaturation	69 (47.3)
Without wheeze at end point	22 (15.1)
Tachypnea alone	2 (1.4)
Desaturation alone	8 (5.5)
Tachypnea + desaturation	12 (8.2)
Any signs at end point	140 (95.9)
Non-responders	6 (4.1)

LUNG FUNCTION IN THE TYPICAL WHEEZY INFANT

Since the measurement of lung function in children between about 2 and 6 years of age is very difficult, much of the information on lung physiology in young children who wheeze has been obtained from studies in infants. In most cases no distinction has been made (and may well be impossible) between atopic wheezy infants and non-atopic wheezy infants when studies of lung function have been undertaken. From the very earliest studies of acutely wheezy young infants it has been shown that they have a typical pattern of airways obstruction with hyperinflation. In infants studied during an epidemic of respiratory syncytial virus (RSV) bronchiolitis, Phelan et al[37] found that lung volume measured by plethysmography (V_{tg}) was about twice normal and resistance markedly increased on the third day of admission, but both were basically back to normal by the fourteenth day. Other investigators found a similar increase in lung volume and resistance during acute bronchiolitis but without such rapid resolution.[38]

Almost all clinical studies and studies in which measurements of lung function have been used have failed to show any meaningful improvement in lung function in acute viral bronchiolitis in response to selective β_2-agonists or corticosteroid therapy.[39–41] In one study which did show an improvement in a proportion of infants with proven acute RSV bronchiolitis, Soto et al[42] found that only 15 out of the 50 infants (30%) studied had a clinically significant improvement in lung function with salbutamol. Interestingly, there was no difference in the incidence of a family history of atopic diseases or of eosinophil counts and IgE levels in the infants who responded compared with those who did not. In contrast to the lack of effect of a selective β_2-agonist in acute viral bronchiolitis, at least two studies have shown an improvement in lung function with inhaled adrenaline (epinephrine), which has, of course, both alpha and non-selective beta actions.[43,44] This suggests that airways obstruction in acute bronchiolitis is more likely to be due to edema and mucus impaction in the inflamed airways than to bronchospasm. There appear to be no studies specifically of atopic infants destined to become asthmatics during a first attack of wheezing unrelated to an epidemic of RSV bronchiolitis.

Critical to our understanding of the pathophysiology of the lungs in wheezy infants is the question as to whether the abnormalities in lung function predate and predispose the infant to develop wheezing illness or whether the abnormality of lung function is the result of an insult to the lungs in an otherwise healthy infant. Some years ago, Godfrey et al[45] measured lung function in groups of infants with chronic lung diseases and were surprised to find that in high proportion of infants with recurrent wheezing after bronchiolitis, lung volume was less than expected for an obstructive lung disease. In other infants, such as those with CF, lung volume was increased as expected. At that time the authors concluded that bronchiolitis so altered lung tissue and airway function that the measurement of lung volume by plethysmography was probably underestimated. However, not long after this Martinez et al[30] reported lung function measured before 3 months of age in a cohort of infants who had never yet had any respiratory illness. During the first year of life the risk of an infant developing a wheezing lower respiratory tract illness was 3.7 times greater for those infants whose airway conductance (the reciprocal of resistance) was in the lower third of the group as compared with those whose values before any illness were in the upper two thirds. In a subsequent study they found that infants with recurrent wheezing in the first 3 years of life had poorer lung function (25% lower V'max,FRC) before developing the first episode of wheezing.[46] Subsequently, other studies also found that infants with a reduced premorbid V'max,FRC were more likely to have clinically diagnosed bronchiolitis in the first year of life.[47,48] In a random cohort study of infants in Australia it was found that a small number had airflow limitation at 4 weeks of age,[49] before any respiratory illness. These infants were more often diagnosed as having asthma at 2 years of age than the controls. Subsequently, Turner et al[50] described the follow-up of these infants to 11 years of age. They had an increased incidence of wheezing in the early years with persistent mild BHR and rather lower lung function at 6 years of age, despite being asymptomatic. Atopy and parental asthma were not more common in this group, who would fit the overall picture of non-atopic early wheezers. These studies raise the interesting possibility that, at least in a proportion of wheezy infants, there is reduced lung function which predisposes them to develop a wheezing illness while infants with better lung function do not wheeze when exposed to the same stimulus. No clear distinction has emerged from these studies between the atopic and non-atopic types of wheezing.

BRONCHIAL RESPONSIVENESS IN THE TYPICAL WHEEZY INFANT

In infants with recurrent wheezing during the first year of life measurements have been made of lung function, BHR and the response to treatment, but in most studies no clear distinction was made between atopic and non-atopic subjects. While almost all agree that when the infant is symptomatic, lung function is abnormal with small airways obstruction and hyperinflation, there has been much less agreement as to the presence of BHR in these infants. Some studies using bronchial provocation challenges have suggested that recurrently wheezy infants, and even totally asymptomatic infants, are hyperresponsive,[51–54] but this begs the question of what is normality and, more particularly, of how the dose of an inhaled agent compares when given to an infant, older child or adult. Stick et al[55] elegantly explored this point and showed that, when corrected for the dose reaching the lungs, normal infants were not hyperresponsive. They went on to study recurrently wheezy infants and in these patients they also found no evidence of BHR.[56] While Clark et al[57] believed that all the infants they studied were hyperresponsive, they found no difference between those with and without lower respiratory tract illnesses. Thus, it has not been possible to demonstrate convincingly during infancy that recurrently wheezy infants have the type of BHR found in older children with asthma. This could be due to the fact that the infants studied were heterogeneous and some may have been atopic and theoretically more likely to be hyperresponsive, while others (probably the large majority) were non-atopic or viral-induced wheezers.

Rather similar conclusions have been reached in studies of the effect of treatment on recurrently wheezy infants. Most have failed to show any convincing response to bronchodilators in the young infants with recurrent wheezing.[19,58] Other studies have failed to show any beneficial effect of inhaled corticosteroids on the course of the disease apart from, possibly, a small effect on bronchial responsiveness.[59,60] On the other hand, occasionally a young wheezy infant does respond in a classical fashion to treatment as if it had asthma, with a substantial improvement in lung function in response to bronchodilators, corticosteroids or both, and there can be little doubt that such an infant is indeed asthmatic.

PROGNOSIS OF ALTERED LUNG FUNCTION IN THE TYPICAL WHEEZY INFANT

For those wheezy infants who become classical asthmatic children, lung function during childhood reflects the severity of their asthma. In those infants who appear to 'grow out' of their wheezing, their lung function and BHR also improve.[61] In a cohort of infants with clearly defined RSV-induced bronchiolitis, Pullan and Hey[62] showed that the very large majority became symptom free, and when lung function was investigated at 10 years of age it was basically normal, with a small proportion of children showing mild BHR. Subsequent studies have largely confirmed these original observations,[63-65] suggesting that most infants with proven viral-induced wheeze in early infancy have an excellent chance of losing all symptoms and having normal lung function in later childhood. There is a tendency to persistent BHR, which may indicate that the original viral infection caused some mild permanent changes in the airways. Interestingly, in the Australian cohort study, the asymptomatic infants with airflow limitation at 4 weeks of age showed increased bronchial responsiveness at 9 months of age (and subsequently at 6 and 11 years of age), which the investigators believe to be related to the reduced lung function, although whether this was intrinsic or acquired has not been established.[50]

LUNG FUNCTION IN THE ATYPICAL WHEEZY INFANT

A number of different disorders can cause wheezing but there have been few if any systematic studies of lung function in young children with such problems. In all these disorders the wheeze is due to airflow limitation at some point in the respiratory tract, which also causes changes in lung function. In the typical wheezy infant, airways obstruction always involves the smaller airways, as it does in some with atypical wheezing due to CF, primary ciliary dyskinesia (PCD) or bronchiolitis obliterans. In some types of atypical wheezing the obstruction is chiefly or entirely in the larger airways, as in compression by a vascular ring or tracheomalacia. Changes in lung compliance are not a feature of the usual types of wheezing disorders since the site of pathology is primarily in the airways and not in the lung tissue, but in wheezing secondary to congenital heart disease there may be a marked reduction in compliance.

Wheezing due to large airway obstruction

In small airways obstruction the forced expiratory F–V curve is always convex with respect to the volume axis, and flow is markedly and progressively reduced as lung

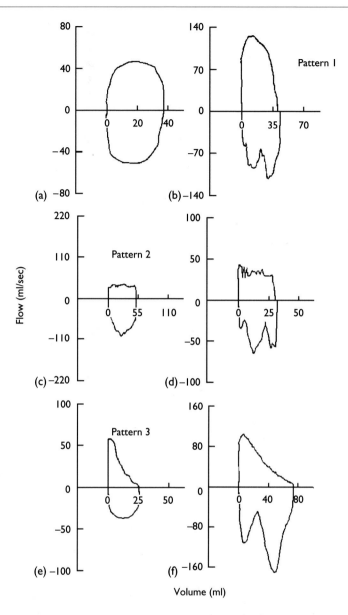

Figure 5.6

Tidal breathing flow–volume (F–V) loop patterns. (a) Normal pattern: round-shaped inspiratory and expiratory limbs. (b) Pattern 1: irregular fluctuations of the inspiratory flow rate (inspiratory fluttering), with normal expiratory shape (associated with laryngomalacia). (c) Pattern 2: flattening of the expiratory limb of the loop with a normal (or variably flattened) inspiratory shape (associated with an airway obstruction between the glottis and mainstem bronchi). (d) Association between expiratory flattening (pattern 2) and inspiratory fluttering (pattern 1) in a child with laryngomalacia and primary tracheomalacia. (e) Pattern 3: early expiratory peak flow followed by reduced flow rates at lower volumes with normal inspiration (associated with reactive airway disease). (f) Association between peripheral airflow limitation (pattern 3) and inspiratory fluttering (pattern 1) in a child with laryngomalacia and asthma. (Redrawn from the data of Filippone et al[68].)

volume is reduced. When the obstruction is in the trachea due to a vascular ring, stenosis or other causes, forced expiratory flow is reduced but the F–V curve tends to lie parallel to the volume axis and flow is much less dependent on volume.[66,67]

Even the pattern of the tidal F–V relationship can indicate the site of obstruction. Filippone et al[68] compared the findings at bronchoscopy with measurements of tidal F–V loops in infants and young children with noisy breathing (Figure 5.6). When the source of the wheeze was in the larynx the inspiratory flow showed fluttering, when the obstruction was in the trachea or main bronchi the expiratory flow was flat with respect to the volume axis and in small airways disease it was convex to the volume axis. Measurements of R_{aw} by plethysmography during tidal breathing can also indicate the site of the obstruction (see Figure 5.5), with resistance rising during inspiration when the obstruction is laryngeal and rising during expiration when it is in the small airways.[28]

Wheezing due to congenital heart disease

From the earliest modern studies of lung function in infants it has been realized that infants with pulmonary engorgement due to congenital heart disease have stiff lungs and reduced compliance,[69,70] changes which may be reversed after corrective surgery.[71] Not only can the lungs be stiff but the abnormal pulmonary vasculature can also impinge on the smaller airways and increase resistance so that the infants wheeze and lung function shows the pattern typical of small airways obstruction (Figure 5.7), In fact, the clinical picture can be dominated by airways obstruction and wheezing rather than heart failure.[72,73] In many such infants the cardiac origin of the problem is not appreciated, especially if a left to right shunt is at atrial rather than ventricular level. Such infants are quite likely to be treated unnecessarily and ineffectively with bronchodilators.[74] Wheezing due to congenital heart disease is far from rare and any infant with wheezing which is in any way atypical should undergo a cardiologic evaluation. In some cases the need for this will only be appreciated when tests of lung function show a reduced compliance in addition to the airways obstruction (Figure 5.8).

Wheezing due to gastroesophageal (GE) reflux

One of the greatest problems in the differential diagnosis of troublesome wheezing in infancy is to distinguish between the infant with the usual type of atopic or non-atopic wheeze and the infant who wheezes because of GE reflux. The clinical and even radiological distinction between these conditions may be very unclear. Some studies have failed to show any clear differences in lung function between infants who wheezed and also had significantly abnormal prolonged esophageal pH recordings as compared with those who wheezed with normal esophageal pH.[75] On the other hand, Sheikh et al[76] found that lung function was less likely to improve after the administration of a bronchodilator in infants with positive esophageal pH studies (16.6%) compared with those with negative studies (66.6%). It must be admitted that in this study the changes were small and the scatter of results was wide. Unfortunately, many typical wheezy

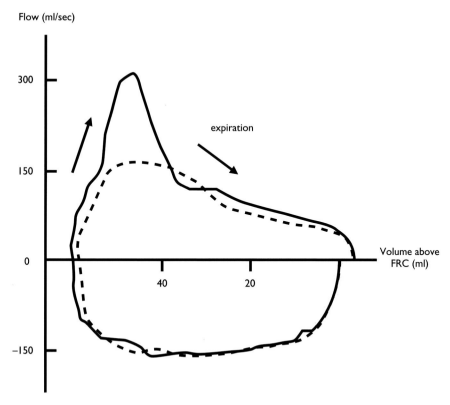

Figure 5.7

Forced expiratory flow–volume (F–V) loop in a 3-month-old infant with a large left to right shunt through an atrial septal defect in whom the cardiac origin of the pulmonary problem only became apparent after the lung function tests were performed. The dashed lines show the tidal F–V loop preceding the forced expiration. (FRC, Functional residual capacity.)

infants do not respond to bronchodilators and therefore failure to respond is not a very helpful indication of GE reflux.

Wheezing due to other types of COPD

There are a number of other conditions which result in COPD in infancy and early childhood besides those causing typical atopic or non-atopic wheezing. Unfortunately, the changes in lung function in these conditions may be identical to those in typical wheezy infants with large and small airways obstruction and hyperinflation. Children with CF may well have normal lung function before their lung disease develops and some show improvement with bronchodilators when lung function is reduced.[77–80] Infants with post-adenoviral bronchiolitis obliterans have a severe type of obstructive

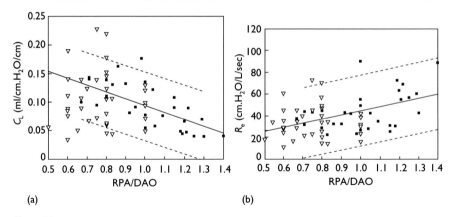

(a)   (b)

Figure 5.8

(a) Relationship between the pulmonary compliance (C_L) corrected for length and the ratio of pulmonary artery to aortic diameter (RPA/DAO) in control infants (open triangles) and infants with left to right shunts (solid squares). (b) Relationship between pulmonary resistance (R_e) and the ratio of pulmonary artery to aortic diameter in control infants (open triangles) and infants with left to right shunts (solid squares). (Redrawn from the data of Yau et al.[73])

lung disease unresponsive to treatment.[81] There appear to be no studies of lung function in infants with PCD.

BRONCHIAL HYPERRESPONSIVENESS IN THE PRESCHOOL CHILD

While the importance of BHR in the wheezy infant is unclear and its role in differential diagnosis is uncertain, there is good evidence that older infants and preschool children who wheeze have BHR[36] and that the nature of the disease influences the type. In older children we have shown that BHR to the inhalation of AMP is far more specific for asthma than is methacholine and that few children with other types of COPD are hyperresponsive to AMP.[82] Using the auscultation (PCwheeze) technique to measure bronchial responsiveness in preschool children, Avital et al[83] compared 39 children with asthma (mean of 4.3 years of age) with 15 children (mean of 4.4 years of age) with other types of COPD. They found that children with asthma responded to both AMP and methacholine while those with COPD only responded to methacholine (Figure 5.9). The intersection point for sensitivity and specificity of AMP for a diagnosis of asthma versus COPD was almost 90% whereas that for methacholine was only 52%. These studies show that wheezy preschool children with asthma are hyperresponsive and that hyperreponsivity to AMP may be used to distinguish between those with asthma and those with other types of COPD. There have not yet been any systematic studies of bronchial responsivity to different stimuli in atopic versus non-atopic or viral-induced wheezers. Failure to show hyperresponsiveness to methacholine should indicate the need to seek a different cause for the wheeze such as large airway obstruction rather than obstruction due to asthma or COPD.

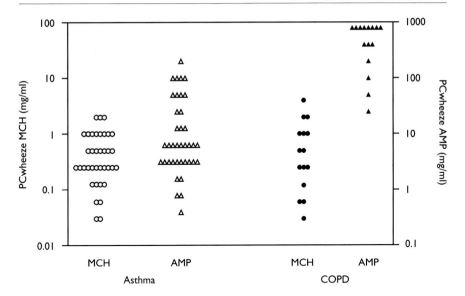

Figure 5.9

Individual results of the provoking dose of methacholine (MCH, circles) and adenosine 5′-monophosphate (AMP, triangles) at the end point of bronchial challenges by the auscultatory method in young children with asthma (open symbols) or other chronic obstructive pulmonary diseases (COPD) (closed symbols). (Redrawn from the data of Avital et al.[83])

IS THERE A PLACE FOR TESTS OF LUNG FUNCTION IN THE WHEEZY INFANT?

While there is no doubt that tests of lung function can be performed in sick infants and tests of bronchial responsivity in preschool children, it is very important to consider whether such tests can make a meaningful contribution to management as they do in older children and adults. Given the difficulty of performing lung function tests in infants, which can only be done under sedation in most cases, it is important to carefully define the situation in which such tests should be recommended. Consideration must be given to the type of test to be used and the risk–benefit relationship in each situation. A review of recent published reports involving the measurement of lung function in infants of all kinds showed that of 62 peer-reviewed studies in the past five years almost 95% were for research purposes and none looked specifically at the place of lung function testing in the management of the infant with a respiratory problem. Just over one fifth of studies involved wheezy babies, again with the very large majority being for research purposes. This is understandable since the management of infants with lung disease cannot advance without adequate information on the way disease affects lung function and how it responds to treatment, especially when new treatments become available. Research is also necessary to develop better tests of lung function and this in turn requires the testing of lung function in healthy infants in order to define the spectrum of normality. In most situations the research will convey little if any benefit on the individual patient and the results are unlikely to materially alter the management of the individual in the short term. Knowledge gained from a clinical trial may improve treatment in the long term.

Given that most investigators using the measurement of lung function in very young children are doing so for research purposes, there are nevertheless at least three situations in which lung function testing could be recommended for the wheezy infant.

The infant with severe continuous COPD

Such infants who do not respond to an adequate clinical trial of combined cortico-steroid and bronchodilator therapy are recommended to undergo lung function testing. There are a number of diseases which can present with this picture, including CF, PCD, bronchiolitis obliterans, GE reflux and congenital heart disease. Before proceeding to tests of lung function, such patients would normally have had a chest radiograph, probably computerized chest tomography, a sweat test, barium swallow, flexible bronchoscopy and echocardiography. Assuming that these have not yielded the correct diagnosis, lung function tests should be performed. In such patients measurements should be made of parameters obtained during forced expiration before and after the inhalation of an adequate dose of short-acting bronchodilator. Measurements should also be made of compliance, preferably by the multiple occlusion technique. The unexpected finding of bronchodilator responsiveness in such an infant would suggest a much more intensive trial of anti-asthma medication, while the finding of reduced compliance would suggest reconsideration of the possibility of congenital heart disease. Severe, unresponsive obstruction may justify proceeding to open lung biopsy in some patients. It is questionable whether lung function tests are less invasive than overnight measurement of esophageal pH, but they are certainly less invasive than open lung biopsy. It may be necessary to repeat the tests after the infant has undergone a therapeutic trial of corticosteroids or other treatment in order to document the response.

The infant with persistent or recurrent wheezing of uncertain severity

In such infants in whom there is the need to justify management decisions by obtaining objective evidence lung function testing may be recommended. The finding of a normal F–V loop in an infant known to have attacks of wheezing strongly suggest that the child has typical atopic or viral related non-atopic wheezing rather than a more serious condition requiring investigation. Lung function tests may be needed to convince the family (or the pediatrician) that their child either does or does not require medication, especially corticosteroids, on a long-term basis. Failure to improve abnormal lung function in a wheezy infant with such medication would be an indication not to continue with this type of treatment at this time. A wheezy infant who does not respond to anti-asthmatic medication may do so later and thus it may be necessary to repeat the tests. It is not necessary to undertake tests of lung function in every typical wheezy infant when the clinical response is obvious and the parents understand and accept the explanations they are offered.

The preschool child with suspected asthma

Bronchial provocation challenges may be recommended in the preschool child in whom the diagnosis of asthma is suspected but not definite, usually young children between the ages of 3 and 6 with unexplained chronic cough. Using surrogates for the measurement of lung function such as the detection of wheezing, mild hypoxia or tachypnea (the PCwheeze method) or by other means, the presence or absence of BHR can be determined. If the provoking agent is AMP, a positive result is highly sensitive and specific for asthma in this age group. Provocation with methacholine is equally sensitive but less specific and is positive in other types of chronic lung disease in early childhood. The role of bronchial challenge tests in young infants is uncertain, as few studies have been performed. The procedure is more complicated in infants since tests of lung function must be used, which need to be repeated with each dose of challenge agent.

If these indications are kept in mind, then infants and preschool children will not be subjected to unnecessary testing of lung function, but for those in whom testing is indicated, the results may make a major contribution to the diagnosis and management of the problem.

REFERENCES

1. Cross KW. The respiratory rate and ventilation in the newborn baby. *J Physiol* 1949; **109**: 459–74.

2. Cross KW, Warner P. The effect of inhalation of high and low oxygen concentrations on the respiration of the newborn infant. *J Physiol* 1951; **114**: 283–95.

3. Cook CD, Sutherland JM, Segal S et al. Studies of respiratory physiology in the newborn infant III. Measurement of mechanics of respiration. *J Clin Invest* 1957; **36**: 440–8.

4. Swyer PR, Wrights JJ. Ventilation and ventilatory mechanics in the newborn. *J Pediatr* 1960; **56**: 612–21.

5. Wallgren G, Geubelle F, Koch G. Studies of the mechanics of breathing in children with congenital heart lesions. *Acta Paediatr* 1960; **49**: 415–25.

6. Stocks J, Sly PD, Tepper RS, Morgan WJ. *Infant Respiratory Function Testing.* (Wiley-Liss: New York, 1996.)

7. Motoyama EK, Laks H, Oh T et al. Deflation flow–volume (DFV) curves in infants with congenital heart disease (CHD): evidence for lower airway obstruction. *Circulation* 1978; **57** (**Suppl ll**): 107.

8. Godfrey S, Bar-Yishay E, Arad I et al. Partial expiratory flow volume curves in infants. *Pediatr Res* 1982; **16**: 690.

9. Taussig LM, Landau LI, Godfrey S, Arad I. Determinants of forced expiratory flows in newborn infants. *J Appl Physiol* 1982; **53**: 1220–7.

10. Godfrey S, Bar-Yishay E, Arad I et al. Flow–volume curves in infants with lung disease. *Pediatrics* 1983; **72**: 517–22.

11. Turner DJ, Stick SM, LeSouef KL et al. A new technique to generate and assess forced expiration from raised lung volume in infants. *Am J Resp Crit Care Med* 1995; **151**: 1441–50.

12. Feher A, Castile R, Kisling J et al. Flow limitation in normal infants: a new method for forced expiratory maneuvers from raised lung volumes. *J Appl Physiol* 1996; **80**: 2019–25.

13. LeSouef PN, England SJ, Bryan AC. Total resistance of the respiratory system in preterm infants with and without an endotracheal tube. *J Pediatr* 1984; **104**: 108–11.

14. Masters IB, Seidenberg J, Hudson I et al. Longitudinal study of lung function in normal infants. *Pediatr Pulmonol* 1987; **3**: 3–7.

15. Springer C, Vilozni D, Bar-Yishay E et al. Comparison of airway resistance and total respiratory system resistance in infants. *Am Rev Resp Dis* 1993; **148**: 1008–12.

16. Olinsky A, Bryan AC, Bryan MH. A simple method of measuring total respiratory system compliance in newborn infants. *S Afr Med J* 1976; **50**: 128–30.

17. Desager KN, Cauberghs M, Naudts J, van de Woestijne KP. Influence of upper airway shunt on total respiratory impedance in infants. *J Appl Physiol* 1999; **87**: 902–9.

18. Rutter N, Milner AD, Hiller EJ. Effect of bronchodilators on respiratory resistance in infants and young children with bronchiolitis and wheezy bronchitis. *Arch Dis Child* 1975; **50**: 719–22.

19. Hayden MJ, Wildhaber JH, LeSouef PN. Bronchodilator responsiveness testing using raised volume forced expiration in recurrently wheezing infants. *Pediatr Pulmonol* 1998; **26**: 35–41.

20. Hall GL, Hantos Z, Wildhaber JH et al. Methacholine responsiveness in infants assessed with low frequency forced oscillation and forced expiration techniques. *Thorax* 2001; **56**: 42–7.

21. Desager KN, Buhr W, Willemen M et al. Measurement of total respiratory impedance in infants by the forced oscillation technique. *J Appl Physiol* 1991; **71**: 770–6.

22. Henry RL, Hodges IGC, Milner AD, Stokes GM. Respiratory problems 2 years after acute bronchiolitis in infancy. *Arch Dis Child* 1983; **58**: 713–16.

23. Frey U, Silverman M, Kraemer R, Jackson AC. High-frequency respiratory impedance measured by forced-oscillation technique in infants. *Am J Resp Crit Care Med* 1998; **158**: 363–70.

24. Dubois AB, Botelho SY, Bedell GN et al. A rapid plethysmographic method for measuring thoracic gas volume: a comparison with a nitrogen washout method for measuring functional residual capacity in normal subjects. *J Clin Invest* 1956; **35**: 322–6.

25. Dubois AB, Botelho SY, Comroe JHJ. A new method for measuring airway resistance in man using a body plethysmograph: values in normal subjects and in patients with respiratory disease. *J Clin Invest* 1956; **35**: 327–35.

26. Stocks J, Godfrey S. Specific airway conductance in relation to postconceptional age during infancy. *J Appl Physiol* 1977; **43**: 144–54.

27. Stocks J, Levy NM, Godfrey S. A new apparatus for the accurate measurement of airway resistance in infancy. *J Appl Physiol* 1977; **43**: 155–9.

28. Beardsmore CS, Godfrey S, Shani N et al. Airway resistance measurements throughout the respiratory cycle in infants. *Respiration* 1986; **49**: 81–93.

29. Godfrey S. TGV or not TGV in WB? That is the question. *Pediatr Pulmonol* 1991; **10**: 73–7.

30. Martinez FD, Morgan WJ, Wright AL et al and the Group Health Medical Associates' Personnel. Diminished lung function as a predisposing factor for wheezing respiratory illness in infants. *N Engl J Med* 1988; **319**: 1112–17.

31. Avital A, Bar-Yishay E, Springer C, Godfrey S. Bronchial provocation tests in young children using tracheal auscultation. *J Pediatr* 1988; **112**: 591–4.

32. Noviski N, Cohen L, Springer C et al. Bronchial provocation determined by breath sounds compared with lung function. *Arch Dis Child* 1991; **66**: 952–5.

33. Springer C, Godfrey S, Picard E et al. Efficacy and safety of methacholine bronchial challenge performed by auscultation in young asthmatic children. *Am J Resp Crit Care Med* 2000; **163**: 857–60.

34. Cockcroft DW, Killian DM, Mellon JJA, Hargreave FE. Bronchial reactivity to inhaled histamine: a method and clinical survey. *Clin Allergy* 1977; **7**: 235–43.

35. Sprikkelman AB, Schouten JP, Lourens MS et al. Agreement between spirometry and tracheal auscultation in assessing bronchial responsiveness in asthmatic children. *Resp Med* 1999; **93**: 102–7.

36. Yong SC, Smith CM, Wach R et al. Methacholine challenge in preschool children: methacholine–induced wheeze

versus transcutaneous oximetry. *Eur Resp J* 1999; **14**: 1175–8.

37. Phelan PD, Williams HE, Freeman M. The disturbances of ventilation in acute viral bronchiolitis. *Aust Paediatr J* 1968; **4**: 96–104.

38. Stokes GM, Milner AD, Hodges IGC, Groggins RC. Lung function abnormalities after acute bronchiolitis. *J Pediatr* 1981; **98**: 871–4.

39. Radford M. Effect of salbutamol in infants with wheezy bronchitis. *Arch Dis Child* 1975; **50**: 535–8.

40. Springer C, Bar-Yishay E, Uwayyed K et al. Corticosteroids do not affect the clinical or physiological status of infants with bronchiolitis. *Pediatr Pulmonol* 1990; **9**: 181–5.

41. Sly PD, Lanteri CJ, Raven JM. Do wheezy infants recovering from bronchiolitis respond to inhaled salbutamol? *Pediatr Pulmonol* 1991; **10**: 36–9.

42. Soto ME, Sly PD, Uren E et al. Bronchodilator response during acute viral bronchiolitis in infancy. *Pediatr Pulmonol* 1985; **1**: 85–90.

43. Sanchez I, DeKoster J, Powell RE et al. Effect of recemic epinephrine and salbutamol on clinical score and pulmonary mechanics in infants with bronchiolitis. *J Pediatr* 1993; **122**: 145–51.

44. Lodrup Carlsen KC, Carlsen KH. Inhaled nebulized adrenaline improves lung function in infants with acute bronchiolitis. *Resp Med* 2000; **94**: 709–14.

45. Godfrey S, Beardsmore CS, Maayan C, Bar-Yishay E. Can thoracic gas volume be measured in infants with airways obstruction? *Am Rev Resp Dis* 1986; **133**: 245–51.

46. Martinez FD, Morgan WJ, Wright AL et al. Initial airway function is a risk factor for recurrent wheezing respiratory illnesses during the first 3 years of life. *Am Rev Resp Dis* 1991; **143**: 312–16.

47. Young S, O'Keeffe PT, Arnott J, Landau LI. Lung function, airway responsiveness, and respiratory symptoms before and after bronchiolitis. *Arch Dis Child* 1995; **72**: 16–24.

48. Dezateux C, Stocks J, Wade AM et al. Airway function at one year: association with premorbid airway function, wheezing, and maternal smoking. *Thorax* 2001; **56**: 680–6.

49. Young S, Arnott J, Le Souef PN, Landau LI. Flow limitation during tidal expiration in symptom-free infants and the subsequent development of asthma. *J Pediatr* 1994; **124**: 681–8.

50. Turner SW, Palmer LJ, Rye PJ et al. Infants with flow limitation at 4 weeks: outcome at 6 and 11 years. *Am J Resp Crit Care Med* 2002; **165**: 1294–8.

51. Tepper RS. Airway reactivity in infants: a positive response to methacholine and metaproterenol. *J Appl Physiol* 1987; **62**: 1155–9.

52. Geller DE, Morgan WJ, Cota KA et al. Airway responsiveness to cold, dry air in normal infants. *Pediatr Pulmonol* 1988; **4**: 90–7.

53. LeSouef PN, Geelhoed GC, Turner DJ et al. Response of normal infants to inhaled histamine. *Am Rev Resp Dis* 1989; **139**: 62–6.

54. Gutkowski P. Airway responsiveness following wheezy bronchitis in infants. *Eur Resp J* 1990; **3**: 807–11.

55. Stick SM, Turnbull S, Chua HL et al. Bronchial responsiveness to histamine in infants and older children. *Am Rev Resp Dis* 1990; **142**: 1143–6.

56. Stick SM, Arnott J, Turner DJ et al. Bronchial responsiveness and lung function in recurrently wheezy infants. *Am Rev Resp Dis* 1991; **144**: 1012–15.

57. Clark JR, Reese A, Silverman M. Bronchial responsiveness and lung function in infants with lower respiratory tract illness over the first six months of life. *Arch Dis Child* 1992; **67**: 1454–8.

58. Lenney W, Milner AD. At what age do bronchodilator drugs work. *Arch Dis Child* 1978; **53**: 532–5.

59. Stick SM, Burton PR, Clough JB et al. The effects of inhaled beclomethasone dipropionate on lung function and histamine responsiveness in recurrently wheezy infants. *Arch Dis Child* 1995; **73**: 327–32.

60. Wong JYW, Moon S, Beardsmore C et al. No objective benefit from steroids inhaled via a spacer, in infants recovering from

bronchiolitis. *Eur Resp J* 2000; **15**: 388–94.

61. Balfour-Lynn L, Tooley M, Godfrey S. Relationship of exercise-induced asthma to clinical asthma in childhood. *Arch Dis Child* 1981; **56**: 450–4.

62. Pullan CR, Hey EN. Wheezing, asthma and pulmonary dysfunction 10 years after infection with respiratory syncytial virus in infancy. *Br Med J* 1982; **284**: 1665–9.

63. Noble V, Murray M, Webb MSC et al. Respiratory status and allergy nine to 10 years after acute bronchiolitis. *Arch Dis Child* 1997; **76**: 315–19.

64. Wennergren G, Amark M, Amark K et al. Wheezing bronchitis reinvestigated at the age of 10 years. *Acta Paediatr* 1997; **86**: 351–5.

65. Sporik R, Holgate ST, Cogswell JJ. Natural history of asthma in childhood – a birth cohort study. *Arch Dis Child* 1991; **66**: 1050–3.

66. Tepper RS, Eigen H, Brown J, Hurwitz R. Use of maximal expiratory flows to evaluate central airways obstruction in infants. *Pediatr Pulmonol* 1989; **6**: 272–4.

67. Thompson AH, Beardsmore CS, Firmin R et al. Airway function in infants with vascular rings: preoperative and post operative assessment. *Arch Dis in Child* 1990; **65**: 171–4.

68. Filippone M, Narne S, Pettenazzo A et al. Functional approach to infants and young children with noisy breathing. Validation of pneumotachography by blinded comparison with bronchoscopy. *Am J Resp Crit Care Med* 2000; **162**: 1795–800.

69. Howlett G. Lung mechanics in normal infants and infants with congenital heart disease. *Arch Dis Child* 1972; **47**: 707–15.

70. Bancalari E, Jesse MJ, Gelband H, Garcia O. Lung mechanics in congenital heart disease with increased and decreased pulmonary blood flow. *J Pediatr* 1977; **90**: 192–5.

71. Baraldi E, Filippone M, Milanesi O et al. Respiratory mechanics in infants and young children before and after repair of left-to-right shunts. *Pediatr Res* 1993; **34**: 329–33.

72. Freezer NJ, Lanteri CJ, Sly PD. Effect of pulmonary blood flow on measurements of respiratory mechanics using the interrupter technique. *J Appl Physiol* 1993; **74**: 1083–8.

73. Yau KI, Fang LJ, Wu MH. Lung mechanics in infants with left-to-right shunt congenital heart disease. *Pediatr Pulmonol* 1996; **21**: 42–7.

74. Pisanti A, Vitiello R. Wheezing as the sole clinical manifestation of cor triatriatum. *Pediatr Pulmonol* 2000; **30**: 346–9.

75. Hampton FJ, MacFadyen UM, Beardsmore CS, Simpson H. Gastro-oesophageal reflux and respiratory function in infants with respiratory symptoms. *Arch Dis Child* 1991; **66**: 848–53.

76. Sheikh S, Goldsmith LJ, Howell L et al. Lung function in infants with wheezing and gastroesophageal reflux. *Pediatr Pulmonol* 1999; **27**: 236–41.

77. Hiatt P, Eigen H, Yu P, Tepper RS. Bronchodilator responsiveness in infants and young children with cystic fibrosis. *Am Rev Resp Dis* 1988; **137**: 119–22.

78. Godfrey S, Mearns M, Howlett G. Serial lung function studies in cystic fibrosis in the first 5 years of life. *Arch Dis Child* 1978; **53**: 83–5.

79. Beardsmore CS, Bar-Yishay E, Maayan C et al. Lung function in infants with cystic fibrosis. *Thorax* 1988; **43**: 545–51.

80. Beardsmore C. Lung function from infancy to school age in cystic fibrosis. *Arch Dis Child* 1995; **73**: 519–23.

81. Teper AM, Kofman CD, Maffey AF, Vidaurreta SM. Lung function in infants with chronic pulmonary disease after severe adenoviral illness. *J Pediatr* 1999; **134**: 730–3.

82. Avital A, Springer C, Bar-Yishay E, Godfrey S. Adenosine, methacholine, and exercise challenges in children with asthma or paediatric chronic obstructive pulmonary disease. *Thorax* 1995; **50**: 511–16.

83. Avital A, Picard E, Uwyyed K, Springer C. Comparison of adenosine 5'-monophosphate and methacholine for the differentiation of asthma from chronic airway diseases with the use of the auscultative method in very young children. *J Pediatr* 1995; **127**: 438–40.

6
The wheezy infant and preschool child: differential diagnosis

---

INTRODUCTION

Wheezing is a very common symptom of lung disease in infants and preschool children. The large majority of such children will have viral-related wheezing either following respiratory syncytial virus (RSV) infection in early infancy or later viral infections, but a minority of infants have an atopic background and the wheezing is more like that seen in older children with asthma. The clinical features of these two common causes of wheezing are described in Chapter 4. There are, however, a number of other conditions that cause wheezing or similar symptoms in this age group, which are unrelated to either atopic or non-atopic wheezing. Some of these conditions resemble the common types of wheezing found in infants and preschool children so closely as to be almost indistinguishable on simple clinical grounds and, consequently, these children are frequently treated with anti-asthmatic medications, often for long periods, before the correct diagnosis is made. This is not only a waste of resources but exposes the child to unnecessary medications, including corticosteroids, while delaying more appropriate treatment. In some cases this may have serious long-term consequences when delayed diagnosis and treatment result in irreversible lung disease. The true incidence of these atypical causes of wheezing is difficult to determine and depends on the mix of patients being seen: in a tertiary referral center the incidence will be greater than in community practice. Last but not least, it is important to remember that children may have more than one disease at the same time and, particularly in countries where tuberculosis is endemic, this should always be considered in a child with respiratory symptoms.

IMPORTANT CONDITIONS WHICH MAY PRESENT AS ATYPICAL WHEEZING

There are a number of important conditions which may present as wheezing in infants and preschool children and which may closely resemble atopic or non-atopic (viral) wheezing. The following describes some of the salient features of those conditions which the pediatrician or pediatric pulmonologist is likely to encounter from time to time. It is convenient to group them according the most likely age at which they present but there is a very wide overlap and these age ranges should only be considered a rough guide.

Newborn and very young infants (0–3 months of age approximately)

Bronchopulmonary dysplasia (BPD)

Although BPD is a disease affecting premature infants who have required intensive care in the neonatal period, in its more severe form it results in chronic obstructive pulmonary disease (COPD) which may persist during the first few years of life. The parents and the physician would normally be fully aware of the origin of the problem but in milder forms of BPD the origin may be forgotten and the child may present as a wheezy infant or preschool child. In the child with BPD the symptoms are essentially continuous, with varying amount of breathlessness, wheeze and cough. The physical examination reveals signs of COPD with hyperinflation, prolonged expiration and expiratory wheezing, which is basically similar to the findings in the typical wheezy child. However, in BPD there is often failure to thrive due to the severity of the condition and essentially no response to bronchodilators or corticosteroids. Unlike the typical wheezy infant or preschool child, the chest radiograph is abnormal, with characteristic changes of widespread irregular hyperinflation and fibrosis (Figure 6.1). Except for the mildest forms of BPD there is some

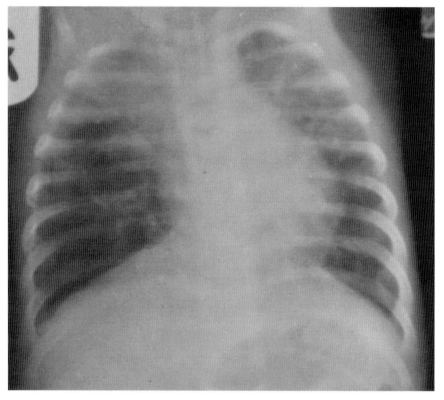

Figure 6.1

Chest radiograph of an infant with bronchopulmonary dysplasia (BPD) showing widespread irregular hyperinflation and fibrosis.

degree of oxygen desaturation. Treatment of BPD is essentially supportive, with added inspired oxygen for those children who are hypoxic, diuretics for those in whom the COPD results in fluid overload and attention to nutrition with the insertion of a feeding gastrostomy if necessary. Many infants with BPD inevitably receive anti-asthmatic medications but the evidence that they do any good is very weak indeed and the overzealous use of corticosteroids merely makes the infant Cushingoid. Taking the clinical, radiological and saturation findings into account, there should be little if any difficulty in distinguishing BPD from the usual type of wheezy infant and preschool child.

Congenital anomalies of the laryngeal region

Lesions producing obstruction of the airway in the region of the larynx essentially cause inspiratory stridor, which should be easy to distinguish from typical small-airway expiratory wheezing. However, parents are often unable to distinguish the timing of the abnormal sound and, in any case parental description of abnormal respiratory sounds often differ widely from those of a physician.[1] The most common laryngeal problem in early infancy is congenital laryngeal stridor in which the supportive structures of the larynx are lax and the arytenoid cartilages get drawn into the laryngeal orifice during inspiration (Figure 6.2), producing the stridor.[2] In the infant with the usual mild to moderate type of congenital laryngeal stridor the child thrives normally and the condition disappears after about

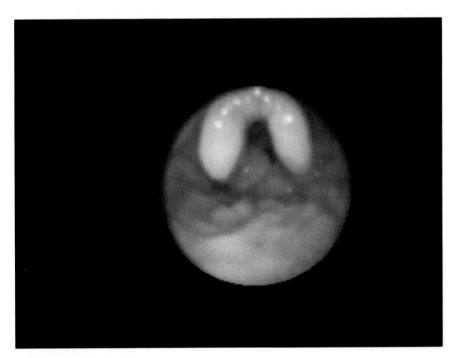

Figure 6.2

Bronchoscopic view of the larynx of an infant with laryngomalacia showing the indrawing of the arytenoid cartilages during inspiration.

18 months. The parents, and sometimes their physician, may well become anxious because of the stridor and this is a good indication to make a definitive diagnosis by bronchoscopy. In more extreme cases there may be failure to thrive because the infant has difficulty in nursing. Occasionally, the problem may be due to paralysis of one or both vocal cords, which can occur in isolation and often recovers spontaneously, or it may be associated with neurological or cardiac anomalies. Subglottic stenosis usually occurs as a result of damage to the airway during resuscitation or intubation, while very rarely the laryngeal region may be obstructed by a cyst or tumor, particularly by a hemangioma. Severe or even life-threatening laryngeal obstruction may occur in infants with subglottic stenosis, cysts or hemangiomas. The location of the obstruction and its distinction from the usual type of wheezing in infancy should be obvious clinically but a definitive diagnosis is best made by bronchoscopy that defines the site and severity of the problem. Treatment depends on the nature of the lesion, with more severe types of obstruction requiring surgery. Medications have no place in the management of these obstructive lesions of the laryngeal region except for hemangiomata for which corticosteroids can be effective.

Congenital anomalies of the trachea and large airways

Unlike the congenital anomalies of the laryngeal region, which usually cause well-defined stridor, lesions lower down in the trachea and large airways can easily be confused with the wheezing heard in the typical wheezy infant. Careful examination may indicate that the abnormal noise is heard more centrally than over the lung fields, and that it is often both inspiratory and expiratory with a much coarser quality than in small-airway disease. When the airway abnormality causes only mild or moderate obstruction the infant thrives and the only problem is the noisy breathing. Sometimes there is superimposed infection if normal ciliary clearance is impeded and there is accumulation of secretions. These infants are very frequently confused with the usual type of wheezy infant and almost inevitably will have received anti-asthmatic medication, often for prolonged periods, before the correct diagnosis is made. Weakness of the supporting rings of cartilage causing tracheomalacia or bronchomalacia may occur in isolation but are often associated with various types of vascular compression.[3] Infants with tracheoesophageal fistula have some degree of tracheomalacia at the site of the fistula, and pooling of secretions with noisy breathing is often the major problem after repair of the defect. In some types of vascular compression of the airway there is a right-sided aortic arch which may be seen even on a plain chest radiograph. The presence of such an anomaly in a wheezy infant should raise the suspicion of airway compression. On the whole, plain chest radiographs are very poor for evaluating airway patency or compression and a computerized tomography (CT) scan is not much better because it is impossible to observe the airway dynamics. While a barium esophagogram may show the presence of an abnormal vessel (Figure 6.3a), the only way of evaluating the severity of the airway compression is by bronchoscopy (Figure 6.3b). Ultimately, a CT scan with contrast may be needed if surgical treatment is being considered. While there is fairly general agreement that surgery is indicated for complete vascular rings because the compression of the airway is likely to increase as the child grows, there is less agreement with other types of compression. If the child is thriving and the airway obstruction is mild to moderate, a conservative policy

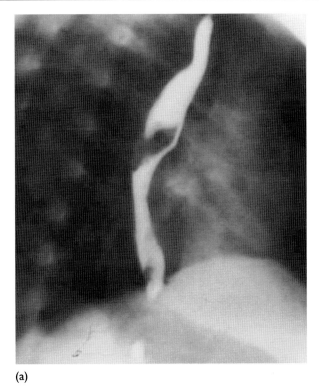

(a)

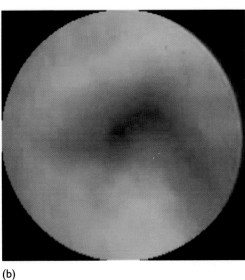

(b)

Figure 6.3

(a) Barium esophagogram from a wheezy infant showing indentation of the esophagus due to compression from behind by an aberrant vessel. (b) Bronchoscopic view of the trachea of another infant with a double aortic arch causing major narrowing of the trachea.

is reasonable, while if it is more severe or if the child is not thriving, surgery is indicated. It is not uncommon for symptoms to persist after surgery, often for a considerable time.[4] Isolated tracheomalacia or bronchomalacia is more problematic and there are no completely accepted treatments. In milder cases a conservative policy is indicated, especially with isolated bronchomalacia (usually on the left) where spontaneous resolution often occurs over a number of years. When tracheomalacia causes severe or even life-threatening episodes of airway obstruction, various surgical techniques can be tried such as aortopexy (pulling the trachea forward by suturing the aorta to the sternum), various reconstructive techniques or the insertion of an airway stent.

Older infants (3–12 months of age approximately)

Croup

Respiratory distress with inspiratory stridor, usually due to a viral infection, which produces laryngitis or laryngotracheabronchitis is usually called croup and is common in the first and second years of life. In one series some 15% of all infants suffered from this type of problem during the first three years of life.[5] Parents (and sometimes doctors) are often unable to clearly distinguish between inspiratory stridor and wheezing, so many infants with croup are thought to be the usual type of wheezy infant. The situation is complicated by the fact that some children with croup do indeed wheeze at the same time. These children have symptoms much like the typical viral-induced wheezing of infancy and the offending agent is often RSV. On the other hand, those with croup unassociated with wheeze are more likely to be infected with parainfluenza virus and less likely to wheeze in later childhood.[5] Some children with croup have recurrent attacks and this is particularly difficult to distinguish from the recurrent attacks of the typical wheezing of infancy and early childhood. While some studies have suggested that children with recurrent croup are more likely to be atopic and have bronchial hyperresponsiveness (BHR),[6,7] this has not been the case in all studies. It is possible that failure to distinguish between isolated croup and croup with wheeze has resulted in some confusion as to the nature of recurrent croup. The distinction between simple croup and the usual wheezing of infancy is not purely academic since management is different. Most infants with croup are worse during the night and the condition resolves spontaneously after one or two nights. In more severe croup, especially if the infant is unable to feed normally, improvement can be hastened by systemic corticosteroids.[8] Acute benefit can also be obtained by nebulized inhaled corticosteroids such as budesonide, but at considerably greater cost.[9] Inhalations of epinephrine (adrenaline) improve the obstruction by reducing mucosal edema while selective β-agonists are not effective in croup since the problem is not bronchospasm. In the infant or young child with typical croup there is no indication for the use of other anti-asthmatic medications or for prophylactic treatment. The management of recurrent croup is problematic and it is far from certain that prophylactic medication is either effective or indicated.

Gastroesophageal reflux (GER)/aspiration

Regurgitation of feeds is not at all uncommon in the first year of life but most infants grow out of this problem over the following months. Subsequently, respiratory illnesses are not more common when compared with control infants.[10] On the other hand, GER can be

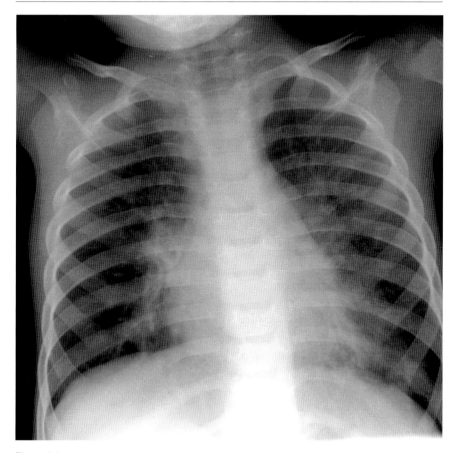

Figure 6.4

Chest radiograph of a wheezy infant showing hyperinflation and also small infiltrates in both lungs.

problematic if excessive or if aspiration of stomach contents into the lungs also occurs. Massive reflux and aspiration produces a dramatic picture due to obstruction of the airway and infection but far more important, in the present context, are repeated small aspirations which cause wheezing and may be extremely difficult to distinguish from the usual types of wheezing of infancy. The chest radiograph of a wheezy infant showing hyperinflation but also some minor infiltrates, almost certainly due to reflux and aspiration, is shown in Figure 6.4. However, such aspirations may be so small that they do not result in significant regurgitation of food at the mouth nor any changes in the chest radiograph. In fact it is not even certain that aspiration has to occur in order to provoke wheezing in children with GER since Cucchiara et al[11] found that GER into the proximal esophagus did not discriminate between patients with reflux disease alone and those with reflux disease complicated by respiratory symptoms. GER can also occur accompanied by respiratory but not gastrointestinal symptoms. In a study of 84 infants with daily wheezing not adequately controlled by anti-asthma medication, Sheikh et al[12] found that of the

54 infants with significant GER on measurement of esophageal pH, 24 (44%) had no gastrointestinal symptoms. With GER the infant may simply develop an attack of respiratory distress with wheezing, hyperinflation and possibly mild hypoxia which resolves spontaneously over a few hours. The only distinguishing clinical feature from atopic or non-atopic (viral) typical wheezing that we have sometimes noted is that the onset and recovery from the attack can be much more sudden. In the study of Sheikh et al[12] measurements of lung function showed that wheezy infants with or without reflux had small-airways obstruction but fewer of those with GER responded to a bronchodilator.

The correct diagnosis may only be reached by a process of exclusion in which no other cause of the symptoms is found together with evidence suggesting that significant GER is present. Once the suspicion of GER and aspiration is raised, the appropriate investigations include a barium study of the swallowing mechanisms and upper gastrointestinal tract, scintigraphy of the stomach and esophagus after a feed of isotopically labeled milk, and bronchoalveolar lavage (BAL) seeking evidence of an increase in fat-containing macrophages (Figure 6.5). Unfortunately, none of these tests are very reliable[13,14] and it is quite unusual for clear-cut evidence of GER and aspiration to be found. Overnight or 24-hour esophageal pH monitoring is the current gold standard for detecting an abnormal degree of GER[15] but the proof of abnormal GER is not proof of aspiration. When there is a real suspicion that the wheezing is due to GER and aspiration, a clinical trial of antacid and anti-reflux treatment is indicated, and the beneficial effects in carefully conducted

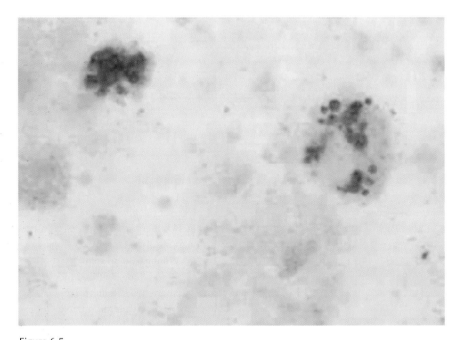

Figure 6.5

Bronchoalveolar lavage (BAL) preparation in an infant with recurrent wheezing and aspiration showing fat globules in alveolar macrophages.

studies have been quite convincing.[16] The real problem is when the suspicion persists but the infant fails to improve with anti-reflux treatment and the only alternative is surgical plication of the gastroesophageal junction. In these infants, the combination of troublesome symptoms, failure to respond to anti-asthmatic and anti-reflux medication, and exclusion of other diagnoses coupled with a high index of suspicion that GER is at the root of the problem will dictate the need for surgery as a last resort.

Cystic fibrosis (CF)

With increasing awareness of the disease and genetic screening, the chances of missing the diagnosis of CF in an infant or young child are decreasing. However, there are families unaware that they carry one of the CF genes and inevitably children are still being born with the disease, which does not always present in such classical ways as meconium ileus or severe chest infections with failure to thrive. One way in which the correct diagnosis may be missed is when CF presents in an infant or young child with troublesome wheezing. Many years ago Lloyd-Still et al[17] described 17 infants with CF under 1 year of age who presented with bronchiolitis and in whom there was a high mortality, partly due to the delay in diagnosis. More recently, Katzelnelson et al[18] described a similar series of infants (15 over a 19-year period) who were treated with large doses of corticosteroids in addition to their treatment for CF and who had a much better prognosis, probably due to the improvement in treatment of CF in the intervening years. They were unable to explain why these infants presented with a bronchiolitic picture and, since affected siblings did not also present in this way, it is unlikely to be genetically linked. There is no doubt that any wheezy infant coming from a family known to have CF genes or any wheezy infant with failure to thrive should be considered as possibly having CF and investigated appropriately. Not all perfectly typical wheezy infants with atopic or non-atopic recurrent wheezing and without failure to thrive should be sent for a sweat test or genotyping, which often generates unnecessary anxiety in the family. Nevertheless, given the very poor prognosis when the diagnosis of CF is missed or delayed and the apparent good response of CF bronchiolitis to corticosteroids, in addition to other measures, such investigations are probably justified in the wheezy infant who has persistent or very troublesome wheezing even in the absence of failure to thrive.

Cardiac anomalies – 'cardiac asthma'

The term 'cardiac asthma' was applied in the past to elderly patients with predominantly left heart failure who had attacks of breathlessness, essentially due to fluid overload in the lungs. However, for quite a number of years it has been realized that infants, too, can develop 'cardiac asthma' with marked small-airways obstruction. Wheezing occurs in infants and young children with congenital heart disease[19] when there is increased pulmonary blood flow or increased resistance to pulmonary venous drainage. This may occur with such conditions as an atrial septal defect, ventricular septal defect and total or partial anomalous venous drainage. The infants present with troublesome wheezing, often of a fluctuating nature, which is frequently confused with the typical wheezing of infancy when the cardiac origin of the problem is not appreciated.[19,20] One reason why the cardiac origin of the problem may be missed is that left to right shunting at the atrial level is often much less obvious clinically than at the ventricular level. Pisanti and Vitiello[21] described a child who presented at 6 months of age with recurrent episodes of wheezing who failed to respond to bronchodilators and corticosteroids and only later was found to have cor triatriatum. The clinical picture was dominated by the respiratory symptoms, which all resolved after the congenital heart disease was corrected surgically at 17 months of age. Even experienced pediatricians, not to mention pediatric cardiologists, may miss an atrial septal defect or patent ductus arteriosus on clinical examination in a child who appears to have troublesome persistent or recurrent wheezing. The mechanism of cardiac asthma in these infants is not entirely clear but appears to be related to increased pulmonary blood flow or obstruction to pulmonary venous return resulting in the congestion of small vessels surrounding the broncheoli. From a functional point of view these infants have both large- and small-airways obstruction and stiff lungs, as shown by an increase in total pulmonary resistance and reduced maximal expiratory flow at low lung volume, together with reduced lung compliance.[22–25] Once the diagnosis is suspected, the infant should be examined by an experienced pediatric cardiologist and echocardiography should be performed. Management consists of making the correct cardiac diagnosis and treating the child appropriately while avoiding anti-asthmatic medication.

Young children (1–6 years of age approximately)

Almost all of the conditions already discussed that can cause wheezing in infants and very young children can also present for the first time in older preschool children, but there are other conditions which more commonly present in this age group.

Foreign-body (FB) aspiration

The sudden onset of persistent symptoms in an otherwise healthy infant or preschool child should raise the suspicion of the inhalation of a FB, even in a very young child. Personal experience shows that some 14% of FB removed from the lungs are from infants less than 12 months of age and 57% from children between the ages of 1 and 3. Thus, the early preschool years are the commonest age for FB aspiration, especially in boys.[26,27] Most FB aspirated by children are of vegetable origin or parts of plastic toys and are not visible on a chest radiograph. In some cases the diagnosis is obvious and immediate because the child is seen to choke after putting the FB in the mouth; however, in many children the aspiration occur with no adult witness present and without causing any immediate respiratory distress. Such children present later with unexplained respiratory symptoms such as the development of cough, fever or persistent or recurrent pneumonia. On examination, wheezing may be heard which may be unilateral but is often difficult to localize. The onset of wheezing in a child in this age group who has never wheezed before and has no personal or family background of atopy should always raise the possibility of FB aspiration. This is even more likely if there is either localized hyperinflation or atelectasis on the chest radiograph. While screening of the lungs is traditional when looking for evidence of FB aspiration it is often negative and does not exclude the diagnosis. Once the suspicion of FB aspiration has been raised, bronchoscopy should be performed provided there is no other obvious cause for the wheezing or other symptoms (Figure 6.6). In children, the removal of a FB almost always requires rigid, open-tube bronchoscopy and this is the procedure of choice when there is a moderate to high probability of FB aspiration. Where the diagnosis is less obvious, many would undertake flexible bronchoscopy, which is a lesser procedure, and only proceed to open-tube bronchoscopy if a FB is located.[28] It is far better to undertake a bronchoscopy and find that the cause of the symptoms was not FB aspiration than to leave a FB in the lungs, as this can cause irreparable damage and even prove fatal. It should be remembered that in regions where tuberculosis is endemic, endobronchial disease or compression of the airway by tuberculous lymph nodes may mimic typical atopic or non-atopic wheezing or large-airway obstruction due to FB aspiration and produce similar symptoms.[29]

Primary ciliary dyskinesia (PCD; immotile cilia syndrome)

This congenital anomaly of the microtubular structure of cilia in the respiratory tract and elsewhere was originally described in association with bronchiectasis, sinusitis and cardiac situs inversus (Kartagener's syndrome). It is now known that this is only an extreme version of what is not such an uncommon problem. Most children with PCD are much more mildly affected and are very frequently misdiagnosed as asthmatic because the most prominent symptoms are cough and recurrent wheezing with or without pulmonary infections, otitis media and sinusitis.[30] The combination of troublesome upper airway disease and asthma that is poorly, if at all, responsive to treatment should always raise the possibility that the child has PCD. In most cases, overt bronchiectasis only develops in children in whom the correct diagnosis is missed and who do not receive appropriate treatment. In a prospective longitudinal study of a cohort of patients with PCD, Ellerman and Bisgaard[31] found that lung function in those entering the study early as children was better than in those who were diagnosed as adults. The lung function of the children was better preserved [forced expiratory volume (FEV_1) 72% predicted falling to 69% predicted] during the follow-up for some 7 years. Lung function remained stable in most patients during treatment by daily physiotherapy and antibiotics on an as-needed basis according to monthly sputum cultures. The commonest organisms isolated were *Haemophilus influenza*, *Streptococcus pneumoniae* and *Staphylococcus aureus* but, in contrast to patients with CF, *Pseudomonas aeruginosa* was rarely isolated. The diagnosis of PCD depends upon the clinical picture and the demonstration of abnormal ciliary structure and/or function. Brush biopsies from the nasal mucosa are usually adequate to examine for ciliary motility and for ultrastructure by electron microscopy. In our experience, when good ciliary movement is seen on light microscopy it is rare to find any abnormality on electron microscopy. Management of PCD depends upon preventing progressive lung and sinus disease by the use of physiotherapy and appropriate antibiotics and sinus drainage if necessary. Some children seem to benefit from the inhalation of a bronchodilator but corticosteroids and other anti-asthmatic medications are of no value. In correctly managed children the prognosis is good, although male sterility is the rule.

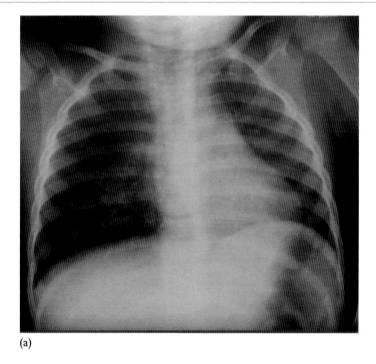

(a)

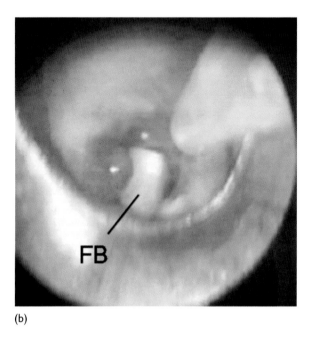

(b)

Figure 6.6

(a) Chest radiograph showing hyperinflation of the right lower lobe in an infant with noisy breathing initially thought to be due to asthma. (b) Bronchoscopic view of the foreign body (FB) lying in the right main bronchus which was causing the wheezing.

Bronchiolitis obliterans

One of the most difficult management problems in children is COPD which can develop following viral pneumonia, especially adenoviral pneumonia.[32] The children are usually very ill during the adenoviral infection, with systemic as well as pulmonary involvement, and after recovery from this initial episode many continue to be troubled by persistent wheezing and breathlessness, which can be disabling. Inevitably, the children are thought to be asthmatic and treated with anti-asthmatic medications, including corticosteroids, but there is no evidence of any useful response to such treatment.[33] Except by chance, they do not have a personal or family background of atopic disease and in studies of bronchial responsiveness in those old enough to be investigated, unlike asthmatic children, they are not hyperresponsive to the inhalation of adenosine 5′-monophosphate (AMP).[34] The diagnosis can only be made on the basis of clinical observation, the appearance of areas of 'ground glass' changes on the chest CT scan, the exclusion of other causes of chronic wheezing, and failure to respond to anti-asthmatic treatment. Open lung biopsy is necessary to make a pathological diagnosis of bronchiolitis obliterans but this can rarely be justified on clinical grounds in small children. In some children the disease appears to affect one lung much more than the other and this can eventually lead to a small, hyperlucent lung typical of the Swyer–James syndrome.[35–37] Similar clinical manifestations due to bronchiolitis obliterans can occur after bone marrow or solid organ transplantation. This is a major cause of morbidity and mortality after lung transplantation but this origin of the disease is unlikely to pose any diagnostic difficulty.[38]

Congenital lung/airway anomalies

While most congenital anomalies producing wheezing or noisy breathing would be expected to present during the first weeks or months of life, there are some which only present later because they do not cause early symptoms severe enough to bring the child to the attention of a physician. Isolated bronchomalacia unrelated to vascular compression, usually affecting the beginning of the left main bronchus and often associated with pectus excavatum,[39,40] may present as persistent or recurrent wheezing in the preschool child. Despite the unilateral obstruction, the wheeze may appear to be generalized but careful examination should indicate reduced breath sounds on the affected side. This sign may be wrongly attributed to mucus plugging in asthma, as may the localized hyperinflation which is seen on a plain chest radiograph. The combination of pectus excavatum and wheezing should raise the possibility of this diagnosis, which is best confirmed by bronchoscopy (Figure 6.7). In our experience, most children with this condition recover spontaneously during early childhood and the only intervention required is to avoid the unnecessary use of anti-asthmatic medication. Another congenital anomaly which not infrequently presents at this age is congenital lobar emphysema (CLE). While infants with significant CLE usually present very early, children with milder forms of the disease may present much later.[41–43] Again, despite the usually localized nature of the emphysema, the child is often thought to have asthma with generalized wheezing. The true diagnosis is made by a CT scan, although we usually also undertake bronchoscopy to exclude local obstructing lesions of the airway which may

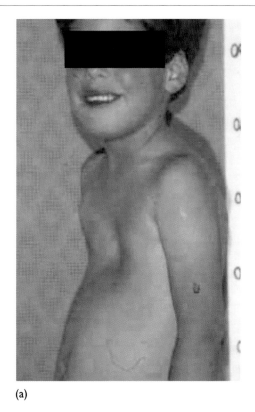

(a)

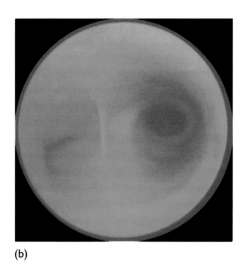

(b)

Figure 6.7

(a) Photograph of a 5-year-old girl with pectus excavatum who had bronchomalacia of the left main bronchus. (b) Bronchoscopic view of the bronchial lesion in another child with the same anomaly.

be amenable to treatment. Management of CLE depends upon the severity of the distress and how it progresses with time.[44] Lobectomy is required in the more severe cases or when the emphysema becomes progressively worse.

WHAT SHOULD AROUSE SUSPICION OF AN ATYPICAL CAUSE OF WHEEZING?

If the correct diagnosis is to be made and treated appropriately, the most important initial step is for the physician to be alert to the possibilities of atypical causes of wheezing and to have a high index of suspicion. The typical types of atopic and non-atopic wheezy infant and preschool child are described more fully in Chapters 3 and 4. Briefly, the infant and preschool child with atopic wheezing usually has a personal or family background of atopic diseases, may begin to wheeze at any time of the year, may have an elevated immunoglobulin E (IgE) level or eosinophilia and may respond reasonably well to anti-asthmatic medications. The non-atopic child with wheeze often has the first attack during the winter RSV epidemic season or attacks only follow presumed viral upper respiratory tract infections. In these children there may or may not be family or personal history of asthma or atopic diseases, the mother may smoke cigarettes, and the infant need not have an elevated IgE level or eosinophilia. The response to treatment is problematic in that most young infants do not respond to anti-asthmatic medication but it is not yet certain that such infants are only from the non-atopic group.

So, what features should raise the suspicion that the infant or preschool child has an atypical cause for the symptoms?

History

There are a number of clues in the history which should raise the possibility that the problem is atypical. However, it should be remembered that what parents describe as abnormal breath sounds may well not mean the same to a physician.[1]

Age of onset of symptoms

The onset of symptoms from birth or shortly afterwards would be very unusual for the typical wheezy infant and should raise the possibility of another cause, particularly congenital anomalies of the airways. Wheezing associated with premature birth, especially if the infant required intensive care, is much more likely to be due to BPD than other causes. The onset of wheezing in an older preschool child may be due to asthma but the possibility of FB aspiration should be considered.

Pattern of attacks

Continuous symptoms with little or no remission is much more likely when the cause of the wheezing is atypical and this pattern should be regarded with great suspicion. Likewise, the sudden onset of symptoms which do not remit is very unlikely in the typical wheezy child and should arouse the suspicion of other causes, particularly FB aspiration.

Relationship to feeding

GER and aspiration are not at all uncommon, especially during the first year of life, in otherwise healthy infants. Aspiration should be considered in the wheezy child who regurgitates or vomits excessively. The infant who coughs and chokes during feeding, or who wheezes afterwards, could have GER but aspiration also occurs during sleep between feeds. Infants with neurological deficits may aspirate during swallowing. Unfortunately, there may be no external manifestations of GER and aspiration in a child with troublesome wheezing and this diagnosis should always be considered in the problematic patient. An 'accidental' form of aspiration can occur if the infant or young child is left to go to sleep lying supine and sucking from a feeding bottle as a comforter. Wheezing due to milk allergy or other types of food allergy is quite uncommon in this age group. Most infants with true milk allergy have dermatological or gastroenterological problems rather than pulmonary disease.[45,46]

Growth and development

Failure to thrive is not a feature of the typical wheezy infant or preschool child and should raise the possibility of an alternative diagnosis. While this is typical of CF, it may also indicate other severe congenital or acquired problems resulting in difficulty in feeding or high energy expenditure.

Family background

A family history of CF or PCD suggests that these diagnoses be considered in the child under investigation for troublesome wheezing. Congenital anomalies of the airways or lungs are not usually familial.

Environmental

Cigarette smoking by parents, especially by the mother, has been clearly associated with an increase of respiratory disease in children and may be the cause of the symptoms when there are no other explanations. Environmental smoking can also exaggerate symptoms in children with asthma. Parents often claim that they never smoke in the home but this is rarely true, and in any case the smell of tobacco persists on their clothing and can adversely affect the child.

Response to previous treatment

It is quite likely that a wheezy infant or preschool child has already received some type of treatment before coming to the attention of the specialist pediatrician or pediatric pulmonologist. The medications include short-term bronchodilators, inhaled or oral corticosteroids and antibiotics. In order to judge the response, it is important to try to determine whether the medication was given in an appropriate dose, by an appropriate route and for an adequate length of time. Failure to show any improvement of symptoms with an adequate dose of bronchodilator or corticosteroid makes the likelihood of atopic wheezing less but does not exclude non-atopic wheezing. It has been suggested that the response to treatment improves with age but this could well be because asthma is more common in the older child while most non-atopic wheezers stop wheezing in early child-hood. Failure to respond to adequate treatment in a cooperative 3–4-year-old child should raise the suspicion that the diagnosis is not asthma.

Examination

There are a number of physical findings on examination which should raise the poss-ibility that the problem is atypical, although even in atypical conditions examination may be entirely normal.

General development

Malnourishment and failure to thrive should not occur in the typical wheezy infant and their presence is strongly suggestive of an alternative diagnosis. Children with psycho-motor retardation may well aspirate on swallowing and this could be the cause of their problem.

Ears and sinuses

Severe or recurrent otitis media or sinusitis occurs in children with PCD.[30]

Shape of the chest

Apart from generalized hyperinflation during an attack, the shape of the chest should be normal in the typical wheezy child. Pectus carinatum suggests severe and chronic hyper-inflation which would be unusual in the typical wheezy infant or preschool child. Skeletal abnormalities such as pectus excavatum may be associated with congenital anomalies of the airway,[40] as may other types of chest deformity or asymmetry.

Breath sounds

Inequality of breath sounds between the two sides is an important sign which may indi-cate a localized cause of airways obstruction or congenital anomaly of lung tissue. While a mucus plug can reduce breath sounds locally in the usual types of wheezy infant and preschool child, persistent inequality of breath sounds between the lungs or between the upper and lower lobes of one lung should be treated very seriously. Even so, an FB or other obstructive lesion may well not reduce airflow enough to be detectable clinically and the presence of equal air entry does not exclude atypical causes of wheezing.

Wheeze and stridor

Continuous abnormal (adventitious) breath sounds heard only during inspiration, espe-cially if monophonic rather than polyphonic, are unlikely to come from the small airways and are much more likely to be recognized as stridor and arise in the larynx or trachea. Localized wheeze heard over one lung or lobe, if persistent, strongly suggest an atypical cause such as bronchomalacia or FB aspiration. Coarse wheezing, which may be both inspiratory and expiratory (unfortunately called 'rhonchi' in current acoustic terminology), heard mainly over the trachea is characteristic of congenital anomalies such as tracheomalacia. Snoring and very coarse stridor-like sounds originate in the nose or nasopharynx and can easily be confused with coarse wheezing but do not have the characteristic musical polyphonic quality heard in the typical wheezy infant or preschool child.

Crackles and other sounds

Crackles or crepitations are discontinuous adventitious sounds which are caused by the sudden opening of many small airways when viscous forces are overcome. They are characteristic of fluid in the airways and, although heard during acute viral bronchiolitis, they are not usually present in the uncomplicated typical wheezy infant. Their presence locally suggests local pathology which requires investigation, even if the child also has generalized wheezing. Transient coarse crackles can originate in the trachea and pharynx and may simply be due to failure to clear normal secretions.

Abnormal heart sounds

Infants with large right to left shunts or raised pulmonary venous pressure may wheeze and the cause can easily be overlooked unless the cardiac condition is recognized. Careful attention should be paid to any abnormal heart sounds or any other cardiac anomalies.

Simple investigations

Most children with problematic recurrent wheezing will often have undergone a number of simple investigations. These will usually include a plain chest radiograph, measurement of oxygen saturation by pulse oximetry, a blood count and possibly measurements of total IgE and eosinophils. Some may have also undergone skin testing with common allergens or the measurement of specific IgE by RAST. These simple investigations may help to alert the physician to the possibility that the problem is atypical.

Chest radiography

Unilateral or localized hyperinflation or atelectasis are strongly indicative of local pathology and require investigation. The large majority of FB aspirated by young children are radiolucent but produce changes on the radiograph when large enough to obstruct an airway. Small local atelectases or infiltrates secondary to mucus plugging may also occur in the child with typical wheezing. Any abnormality of the cardiac outline, such as the presence of a right aortic arch, may suggest a vascular ring or aberrant vessel. Significant infiltrates, recurrent pneumonia or bronchiectasis do not occur in the typical atopic or non-atopic wheezy infant or preschool child and require further investigation.

Oxygen saturation

Pulse oximetry is now widely available and the correct measurement of oxygen saturation is an important simple ancillary investigation. Saturation should be normal in the typical wheezy infant or preschool child apart from during a severe attack. If saturation is persistently reduced this may indicate parenchymal lung disease or cardiac disease as the cause of the wheezing.

IgE measurement and other laboratory tests

Markers of allergy such as an elevated IgE level, eosinophilia, positive skin tests or RAST may be absent in young children with typical wheezing but should raise the possibility of an atypical cause in the older preschool child with troublesome wheezing.

WHEN SUSPICION OF ATYPICAL WHEEZING IS AROUSED WHAT TOOLS ARE AVAILABLE TO HELP WITH DIAGNOSIS?

Once the possibility is raised that the cause of the recurrent wheezing is not the typical atopic or non-atopic wheezing of infancy and early childhood, it is obligatory to undertake relevant further investigations in order to arrive at the correct diagnosis and treatment. The investigations used will depend upon the most likely diagnosis and it is especially important in young children to pay careful attention to the risk–benefit relationship of the investigation. Some of the indications and uses of various investigative procedures in the atypical wheezy infant or preschool child are summarized in Table 6.1.

Radiology

It goes without saying that a plain chest radiograph with both postero-anterior and lateral projections is essential for the investigation of the child with atypical wheeze since clinical examination is an imprecise tool. When FB aspiration is suspected it is traditional to request fluoroscopy or the comparison of inspiratory and expiratory plain films, although we have found these to be of little value and a negative result does not exclude the presence of an FB. CT scans, including recent advances in imaging and contrast enhancement, are now the mainstay of the visualization of many parenchymal lung lesions but are not particularly useful in the visualization of the airways. A CT scan is, of course, very useful in defining the extent of bronchiectasis in children with CF or PCD. CT scans can also be helpful in demonstrating the true nature and extent of vascular rings. These may often be suspected by finding airway compression on a simple barium esophagogram but this does not usually fully define the anomaly. A plain radiograph or CT of the mid-face region may be indicated in children suspected of having chronic sinusitis due to PCD.

Bronchoscopy – BAL

With the advent of flexible fiber-optic bronchoscopes suitable for small children it has become possible to easily identify the cause of atypical wheezing in many infants and young children on an ambulatory basis using brief anesthesia or deep sedation.[47] Instead of guessing whether or not there is tracheomalacia or airway compression, and to what extent it narrows the airway, it is possible to visualize the problem directly with minimal

Table 6.1 Relative value of investigations in the infant and preschool child with some types of atypical wheezing (infant lung function tests are discussed more fully in Chapter 5)

Suspected cause of wheezing	Plain radiograph	Barium swallow	Esophageal pH monitoring	CT scan	Infant lung function	Bronchoscopy/ BAL
Upper airway/larynx	+	–	–	–	–	++++
Trachea/large-airway anomalies	+	++	–	++	+	++++
Lung parenchymal anomalies	++	–	–	++++	+	++
Foreign-body (FB) aspiration	++	–	–	–	–	++++
Reflux and aspiration	++	++	++	–	+	++
Cardiac	+	++	–	+++	+++	++

BAL, Bronchoalveolar lavage; CT, computerized tomography.
Note: A positive bronchial challenge with methacholine in the presence of a negative challenge with adenosine 5'-monophosphate (AMP) suggests one of the above conditions or another atypical cause of wheezing.

risk and disturbance to the child. Bronchoscopy is indicated in almost every infant and preschool child with unexplained wheezing or noisy breathing of an atypical nature in order to determine the site and severity of the abnormality. Noisy breathing in young infants originating in the larynx or subglottic region is often confused with wheezing and the correct diagnosis is easily made by bronchoscopy. Direct inspection of the larynx through the mouth, or even with a flexible laryngoscope, can miss the true cause of the symptoms and we always prefer to use a broncoscope to inspect the trachea and large airways in addition to the larynx. We have seen many instances of laryngeal or tracheal lesions, including hemangiomas, which were erroneously treated as asthma before being referred for bronchoscopy. FB aspiration is particularly important in the differential diagnosis of atypical wheezing in the young child. While the correct procedure for removal of an FB in a young child is rigid open-tube bronchoscopy, in children where the diagnosis is uncertain, flexible fiber-optic bronchoscopy is indicated. If an FB is found, it is then removed by open-tube bronchoscopy.[28] GER with aspiration is an important cause of wheezing in early childhood and notoriously difficult to diagnose. BAL performed during fiber-optic bronchoscopy is informative in patients where aspiration is associated with a high proportion of alveolar macrophages containing large amounts of lipid.[48] Bronchoscopy in trained hands is a safe and painless procedure and should never be the last resort in the investigation of atypical wheezing.

Reflux and aspiration studies

When GER with aspiration is suspected as the cause of atypical wheezing, the diagnosis is usually based on a combination of clinical findings and laboratory tests, since no one test is adequately sensitive and specific. A barium study of swallowing and the upper gastrointestinal tract is usually indicated to determine whether there is aspiration during swallowing or whether there is reflux with or without aspiration into the lungs. Some investigators use radioisotopic-labeled milk with intermittent scanning over the next few hours to seek evidence of reflux and aspiration, but this technique is not particularly sensitive.[14] Since reflux and aspiration may well be intermittent and not present during the barium study, an overnight or 24-hour measurement of esophageal pH is helpful in determining the number and severity of the reflux episodes, although it cannot confirm that aspiration also occurs. BAL to determine the presence of fat-laden alveolar macrophages is the third technique used to investigate this difficult problem.

Infant lung function tests and tests of bronchial responsiveness

Lung function tests in wheezy infants and preschool children are discussed in Chapter 5. Even in specialized infant lung function laboratories these tests are tedious to perform and are only really applicable to infants under about 12–18 months of age who can still be investigated using mild sedation. Apart from research, there are at least three situations in which lung function testing should be considered for purely clinical reasons in the wheezy infant.

- The infant with severe, continuous chronic obstructive lung disease who does not respond to an adequate clinical trial of combined corticosteroid and bronchodilator therapy, and in whom chest radiograph, CT scans, a sweat test, barium swallow and echocardiography are unhelpful. The unexpected finding of bronchodilator responsiveness in such an infant would suggest a much more intense trial of anti-asthmatic medication, while the finding of reduced compliance would suggest reconsideration of the possibility of a congenital heart disease. Severe, unresponsive obstruction may justify proceeding to open lung biopsy in some patients.

• The infant with persistent or recurrent wheezing of uncertain severity for whom there may be the need to justify management decisions. The finding of a normal flow–volume loop between attacks in an infant with documented attacks of wheezing strongly suggests that the child has typical wheezing. Lung function tests may be needed to convince the family (or the physician) that the child either does or does not require medication, especially corticosteroids, on a long-term basis.

• The preschool child in whom the diagnosis of asthma is suspected but not definite, usually young children in the 3–6-year-old age group with unexplained chronic cough. Bronchial provocation challenges can be helpful in making the correct diagnosis. If the provoking agent is AMP, a positive result is highly sensitive and specific for asthma in this age group.[49,50] Provocation with methacholine is equally sensitive but less specific and if positive when the response to AMP is negative, there is a clear indication to seek atypical causes for the symptoms.

Nasal cilia biopsy

In the atypical wheezy infant and preschool child in whom PCD is suspected it is quite easy to perform a nasal brush biopsy with topical anesthesia to see if there are beating cilia under light microscopy. It is usual to send the specimen for examination by electron microscopy but in our experience, and that of others, if beating cilia are seen under light microscopy, then the ciliary ultrastructure is very likely to be normal. The absence of beating cilia on light microscopy does not necessarily imply that the child has PCD.[51]

Echocardiography

Because unrecognized congenital heart disease can present as troublesome wheezing, infants and preschool children with an atypical pattern of wheeze should be examined by an experienced pediatric cardiologist and echocardiography should be performed. Evidence should be sought of increased pulmonary blood flow, pulmonary hypertension or pulmonary venous obstruction. Echocardiography may also define some types of aberrant large vessels and vascular rings compressing the airway and causing wheeze. Angiography is rarely indicated now since a CT scan with contrast can obtain the same information.

Bronchial and lung biopsies

In adults with difficult asthma, bronchial biopsies have been used to determine whether the mucosal pathology is typical of asthma and this approach has recently been suggested for children.[52] Since this normally requires open-tube bronchoscopy, in small children it is not a procedure to be undertaken lightly. There can be few indications for lung biopsy in wheezy infants and preschool children but occasionally lung biopsy is indicated to distinguish bronchiolitis obliterans from other causes of wheezing and to allow more rational management.

CONCLUSIONS

There are a considerable number of conditions which can present as wheezing in the infant and preschool child, which resembles the usual types of atopic or non-atopic (viral-related) wheezing. Many of these infants and children are misdiagnosed and wrongly treated as asthmatics and, in some circumstances, this can result in serious consequences. The pediatrician should be aware of these other conditions and consider them in any infant in whom the wheezing disease is in any way atypical.

REFERENCES

1. Cane RS, Ranganathan SC, McKenzie SA. What do parents of wheezy children understand by 'wheeze'? *Arch Dis Child* 2000; **82**: 327–32.

2. Lis G, Szczerbinski T, Cichocka-Jarosz E. Congenital stridor. *Pediatr Pulmonol* 1995; **20**: 220–4.

3. Valletta EA, Pregarz M, Bergamo-Andreis IA, Boner AL. Tracheoesophageal compression due to congenital vascular anomalies (vascular rings). *Pediatr Pulmonol* 1997; **24**: 93–105.

4. Bakker DAH, Berger RFM, Witsenberg M, Rogers AJJC. Vascular rings: a rare cause of common respiratory symptoms. *Acta Paediatr Scand* 1999; **88**: 947–52.

5. Castro-Rodriguez JA, Holberg CJ, Morgan WJ et al. Relation of two different subtypes of croup before age three to wheezing, atopy, and pulmonary function during childhood: a prospective study. *Pediatrics* 2001; **107**: 512–18.

6. Zach M, Erben A, Olinsky A. Croup, recurrent croup, allergy and airways hyperreactivity. *Arch Dis Child* 1981; **56**: 336–41.

7. Litmanovitch M, Kivity S, Soferman R, Topilsky M. Relationship between recurrent croup and airway hyperreactivity. *Ann Allergy* 1990; **65**: 239–41.

8. Kairys SW, Olmstead EM, O'Connor GT. Steroid treatment of laryngotracheitis: a meta-analysis of the evidence from randomized trials. *Pediatrics* 1989; **83**: 683–93.

9. Godden CW, Campbell MJ, Hussey M, Cogswell JJ. Double blind placebo controlled trial of nebulised budesonide in croup. *Arch Dis Child* 1997; **76**: 155–8.

10. Nelson SP, Chen EH, Syniar GM, Christoffel KK. One-year follow-up of symptoms of gastroesophageal reflux during infancy. Pediatric Practice Research Group. *Pediatrics* 1998; **102**: E67.

11. Cucchiara S, Santamaria F, Minella R et al. Simultaneous prolonged recordings of proximal and distal intraesophageal pH in children with gastroesophageal reflux disease and respiratory symptoms. *Am J Gastroenterol* 1995; **90**: 1791–6.

12. Sheikh S, Goldsmith LJ, Howell L et al. Lung function in infants with wheezing and gastroesophageal reflux. *Pediatr Pulmonol* 1999; **27**: 236–41.

13. Sacco O, Fregonese B, Silvestri M et al. Bronchoalveolar lavage and esophageal pH monitoring data in children with 'difficult to treat' respiratory symptoms. *Pediatr Pulmonol* 2000; **30**: 313–19.

14. McVeagh P, Howman-Giles R, Kemp A. Pulmonary aspiration studied by radio-nuclide milk scanning and barium swallow roentgenography. *Am J Dis Child* 1987; **141**: 917–21.

15. Working Group of the European Society of Pediatric Gastroenterology and Nutrition. A standardized protocol for the methodology of esophageal pH monitoring and interpretation of the data for the diagnosis of gastroesophageal reflux. *J Pediatr Gastroenterol Nutr* 1992; **14**: 467–71.

16. Sheikh S, Stephen T, Howell L, Eid N. Gastroesophageal reflux in infants with wheezing. *Pediatr Pulmonol* 1999; **28**: 181–6.

17. Lloyd-Still JD, Khaw KT, Shwachman H. Severe respiratory disease in infants with cystic fibrosis. *Pediatrics* 1974; **53**: 678–82.

18. Katznelson D, Szeinberg A, Augarten A, Yahav Y. The critical first six months in cystic fibrosis: a syndrome of severe bronchiolitis. *Pediatr Pulmonol* 1997; **24**: 134–6.

19. Cochran ST, Gyepes MT, Smith LE. Obstruction of the airways by the heart and pulmonary vessels in infants. *Pediatr Radiol* 1977; **6**: 81–7.

20. Lister G, Pitt BR. Cardiopulmonary interactions in the infant with congenital cardiac disease. *Clin Chest Med* 1983; **4**: 219–32.

21. Pisanti A, Vitiello R. Wheezing as the sole clinical manifestation of cor triatriatum. *Pediatr Pulmonol* 2000; **30**: 346–9.

22. Motoyama EK, Laks H, Oh T et al. Deflation flow–volume (DFV) curves in infants with congenital heart disease (CHD): evidence for lower airway obstruction. *Circulation* 1978; **57 (Suppl II)**: 107.

23. Freezer NJ, Lanteri CJ, Sly PD. Effect of pulmonary blood flow on measurements of respiratory mechanics using the interrupter technique. *J Appl Physiol* 1993; **74**: 1083–8.

24. Baraldi E, Filippone M, Milanesi O et al. Respiratory mechanics in infants and young children before and after repair of left-to-right shunts. *Pediatr Res* 1993; **34**: 329–33.

25. Yau KI, Fang LJ, Wu MH. Lung mechanics in infants with left-to-right shunt congenital heart disease. *Pediatr Pulmonol* 1996; **21**: 42–7.

26. Banerjee A, Rao KS, Khanna SK et al. Laryngo-tracheo-bronchial foreign bodies in children. *J Laryngol Otol* 1988; **102**: 1029–32.

27. Godfrey S, Springer C, Maayan C et al. Is there a place for rigid bronchoscopy in the management of pediatric lung disease? *Pediatr Pulmonol* 1987; **3**: 179–84.

28. Martinot A, Closset M, Marquette CH et al. Indications for flexible versus rigid bronchoscopy in children with suspected foreign-body aspiration. *Am J Resp Crit Care Med* 1997; **155**: 1676–9.

29. Ahmed A, Mirza S, Rothera MP. Mediastinal tuberculosis in a 10-month-old child. *J Laryngol Otol* 2001; **115**: 161–3.

30. Rossman CM, Newhouse MT. Primary ciliary dyskinesia: evaluation and management. *Pediatr Pulmonol* 1988; **5**: 36–50.

31. Ellerman A, Bisgaard H. Longitudinal study of lung function in a cohort of primary ciliary dyskinesia. *Eur Resp J* 1997; **10**: 2376–9.

32. Murtagh P, Cerqueiro C, Halac A et al. Adenovirus type 7h respiratory infections: a report of 29 cases of acute lower respiratory disease. *Acta Paediatr Scand* 1993; **82**: 557–61.

33. Teper AM, Kofman CD, Maffey AF, Vidaurreta SM. Lung function in infants with chronic pulmonary disease after severe adenoviral illness. *J Pediatr* 1999; **134**: 730–3.

34. Avital A, Springer C, Bar-Yishay E, Godfrey S. Adenosine, methacholine, and exercise challenges in children with asthma or paediatric chronic obstructive pulmonary disease. *Thorax* 1995; **50**: 511–16.

35. Swyer PR, James GC. A case of unilateral pulmonary emphysema. *Thorax* 1953; **8**: 133–6.

36. Cumming GR, MacPherson RI, Chernick V. Unilateral hyperlucent lung syndrome in children. *J Pediatr* 1971; **78**: 250–60.

37. Macek V, Sorli J, Kopriva S, Marin J. Persistent adenoviral infection and chronic airway obstruction in children. *Am J Resp Crit Care Med* 1994; **150**: 7–10.

38. Griese M, Rampf U, Hofmann D et al. Pulmonary complications after bone marrow transplantation in children: twenty-four years of experience in a single pediatric center. *Pediatr Pulmonol* 2000; **30**: 393–401.

39. MacMahon HE, Ruggieri J. Congenital segmental bronchomalacia. *Am J Dis Child* 1969; **118**: 923–6.

40. Godfrey S. Association between pectus excavatum and segmental bronchomalacia. *J Pediatr* 1980; **96**: 649–52.

41. Karnak I, Senocak ME, Ciftci AO, Buyukpamukcu N. Congenital lobar emphysema: diagnostic and therapeutic considerations. *J Pediatr Surg* 1999; **34**: 1347–51.

42. Man DW, Hamdy MH, Hendry GM et al. Congenital lobar emphysema: problems in diagnosis and management. *Arch Dis Child* 1983; **58**: 709–12.

43. Thakral CL, Maji DC, Sajwani MJ. Congenital lobar emphysema: experience with 21 cases. *Pediatr Surg Int* 2001; **17**: 88–91.

44. Eigen H, Lemen RJ, Waring WW. Congenital lobar emphysema: long-term evaluation of surgically and conservatively treated children. *Am Rev Resp Dis* 1976; **113**: 823–31.

45. de Jong MH, Scharp-van der Linden VTM, Aalberse RC et al. Randomised controlled trial of a brief neonatal exposure to cow's milk on the development of atopy. *Arch Dis Child* 1998; **79**: 126–30.

46. Hill DJ, Duke AM, Hosking CS, Hudson IL. Clinical manifestations of cows' milk allergy in childhood. II. The diagnostic value of skin tests and RAST. *Clin Allergy* 1988; **18**: 481–90.

47. Godfrey S, Avital A, Maayan C et al. Yield from flexible bronchoscopy in children. *Pediatr Pulmonol* 1997; **23**: 261–9.

48. Colombo JL, Hallberg TK. Pulmonary aspiration and lipid-laden macrophages: In search of gold (standards). *Pediatr Pulmonol* 1999; **28**: 79–82.

49. Avital A, Bar-Yishay E, Springer C, Godfrey S. Bronchial provocation tests in young children using tracheal auscultation. *J Pediatr* 1988; **112**: 591–4.

50. Avital A, Picard E, Uwyyed K, Springer C. Comparison of adenosine 5'-monophosphate and methacholine for the differentiation of asthma from chronic airway diseases with the use of the auscultative method in very young children. *J Pediatr* 1995; **127**: 438–40.

51. Santamaria F, De Santi MM, Grillo G et al. Ciliary motility at light microscopy: a screening technique for ciliary defects? *Acta Paediatr Scand* 1999; **88**: 853–7.

52. Payne D, McKenzie SA, Stacey S et al. Safety and ethics of bronchoscopy and endobronchial biopsy in difficult asthma. *Arch Dis Child* 2001; **84**: 423–6.

7
Management of wheezing in infants and preschool children

INTRODUCTION

Despite the fact that wheezing in infancy and early childhood is one of the commonest problems seen by the pediatrician, management of these children is often difficult and uncertain. Over the past few years a number of guidelines have been published in order to try to standardize the treatment of asthma in adults and children.[1-4] In these management guidelines it is often tacitly assumed that the very young wheezy child responds in the same way as older children or adults, and although the guidelines suggest minor modifications, they basically recommend the same medication as for older patient with the implication that these are likely to help. The American Academy of Asthma, Allergy and Immunology, in collaboration with the American Academy of Pediatrics and others,[3] published guidelines for managing asthma in children which imply that all infants and young children who wheeze because they are atopic or suffer from viral-induced wheeze may benefit from asthma treatment. Careful reading of the small print in some of the guidelines indicates that all is not as simple as it seems. In the British version there is a warning concerning problems in the management of very young children which emphasizes the difficulty in diagnosis, the fact that most treatments have very poor efficacy and that there are very few controlled trials of treatment in this age group.[2]

In the most recent report from the Global Initiative for Asthma[4] there is a much more cautious approach to the very young child in terms of diagnosis and efficacy of treatment but then the guidelines go on to state (page 132):

> Preschool children and infants. Although there are no well-conducted trials to provide scientific evidence for the proper treatment of asthma *at each step of severity* in these age groups, a treatment algorithm similar to that used in school children is recommended for preschool children and infants.

The italics have been added to show that these most recently amended guidelines also imply that wheezy infants and preschool children have asthma whose severity can be graded as in older children – something that has certainly not been confirmed objectively.

The management of the wheezy infant and preschool child is complicated by the fact that there is considerable uncertainty over the etiology. There are some infants and preschool children with an obvious personal or family background of atopic diseases of whom many, but not all, will go on to develop classical childhood asthma – these children are termed atopic infant or preschool wheezers. Others, probably the large majority, have no personal or family background of atopy or asthma and begin to wheeze as a result of viral infection – these chilren are termed non-atopic infants or preschool wheezers. Evidence suggests that some 80% of wheezy infants and preschool children are in the non-atopic group. It is probable that most of these infants wheeze in response to infections with the respiratory syncytial virus (RSV) or other viruses. Some infants wheeze very transiently (only in the first year or so of life) and these may be infants born with lung function in the lower range of normal in whom the viral infection causes some transient mechanical obstruction of the airways.[5] Others may have recurrent wheezing for several months or years in response to new infections or even non-infectious stimuli because the initial viral infection has damaged the airways and induced a type of bronchial hyperresponsivity. Studies to establish the best management for wheezy infants and preschool children have largely ignored these important differences and 'lumped' all the children together, which may well have masked true differences in response to treatment.

To further complicate management, children with very similar clinical presentations to the typical wheezy infant or preschool child may have totally different problems, such as gastroesophageal reflux, cystic fibrosis or congenital heart disease. The differential diagnosis of this very important group of atypical wheezy infants and preschool children is discussed more fully in Chapter 6. Their management depends upon making the correct diagnosis and then applying the treatment appropriate for the disease. In most cases, medications used for asthma have little or no place in the management of such children, while failure to apply the appropriate treatment may have potentially serious consequences. The reader should consult appropriate texts for the management of these other conditions and these will not be discussed further here.

FIRST TIME WHEEZING IN EARLY INFANCY

The typical wheezy infant presenting for the first time during the winter epidemic season of RSV infections is very likely to be suffering from acute viral bronchiolitis (discussed more fully in Chapter 2). On the other hand, the infant may belong to the group of early transient wheezy infants in whom the attack is likely to be related to a viral infection on a background of reduced lung function, or this may be the first attack in an infant from the atopic group, although this is more likely at an older age. Most of these infants wheezing for the first time neither require nor respond to medications used in asthma and the condition resolves spontaneously in a few days. In those who are more distressed, especially if this interferes with normal feeding or if the infant is hypoxic, active intervention may be needed. Again, apart from oxygen in the hypoxic infant there is little or no evidence that other medications are effective. In particular, it has been shown many times that corticosteroids are of no value in acute viral bronchiolitis. As long ago as 1966, Dabbous et al[6] showed that corticosteroids were ineffective in the treatment of bronchiolitis and by 1970 a report of the American Academy of Pediatrics concluded that there was no scientific basis for the routine administration of corticosteroids in bronchiolitis.[7] Nevertheless, a recent survey undertaken by the European Society for Pediatric Infectious Diseases found > 80% of infants hospitalized with RSV bronchiolitis were given corticosteroids.[8] The situation with respect to sympathomimetic broncho-dilator therapy in wheezy infants is similar, in that most objective studies carried out over a number of years have failed to show any benefit, either clinically or in terms of lung function.[9–11] In some, but not all, studies an improvement has been found using an anticholinergic bronchodilator.[12] Rather more encouraging are a number of recent studies showing an improvement either clinically[11] or physiologically[13,14] in infants with acute bronchiolitis treated with epinephrine (adrenaline). Since selective β_2-agonists given by inhalations are very unlikely to have any adverse effects and are occasionally helpful, it seems reasonable to try this treatment in the first-time wheezy infant who is distressed or whose parents need to be reassured that something is being done.

RECURRENT WHEEZING IN INFANCY AND EARLY CHILDHOOD

As many as 40% of typical wheezy infants have recurrent wheezing during infancy and early childhood, although this is very rarely continuous and therefore unremitting wheezing should raise the possibility of an alternative diagnosis. In some typical wheezy infants the wheezing is related to recurrent viral infections, including reinfection with RSV, while others are atopic children in whom wheezing may be more related to allergy. However, even in the atopic infant it often appears that the wheezing episode is pro-voked by a viral upper respiratory tract infection. The management of the recurrently wheezy infant or preschool child depends upon making the correct diagnosis, excluding atypical causes of wheezing and then determining which, if any, medication is indi-cated. A very important part of management concerns explaining the nature of the problem to the parents so they do not have any false expectations about the efficacy of treatment nor undue worry about the future health of their child. When medications are to be tried, it is essential to keep the age of the patient in mind and assess the ability of the family and the infant to accept the treatment which is being offered.

MAKING THE CORRECT DIAGNOSIS OF RECURRENT WHEEZING

When the infant or preschool child with recurrent wheezing presents for the first time it is important to take a careful personal family history and examine the child fully. The clinical features associated with the typical wheezy infant or preschool child and the dif-ferential diagnosis of other causes of wheezing are discussed more fully in Chapters 4 and 6. The following is a résumé of some of the essential points to bear in mind when making the diagnosis.

- The typical infant with recurrent wheezing following RSV bronchiolitis will usually have had the first attack during a winter epidemic and usually within the first six months of life. A personal or family history of asthma or other allergic diseases are no more common in these children than in other children.

- The typical infant with an atopic background may begin to wheeze or cough at any age, often within the first year of life, but not always related to the winter RSV season. There is often a personal or family history of asthma or other allergic diseases.
- The typical infant with recurrent wheezing related to recurrent viral infections will have repeated attacks of wheezing or coughing associated with other signs of viral infection with little or no problem between attacks.
- Continuous symptoms and failure to thrive are not features expected in the typical wheezy infant or preschool child and should raise the suspicion of other, potentially serious, causes of atypical wheezing.
- As with asthmatic children, cough is a common symptom in typical wheezy infants and preschool children, and parents may well complain that their child coughs, especially at night, and not even notice the wheeze.
- Physical examination is not very helpful in the typical wheezy infant and the child may be completely well between attacks. However, if the abnormal breath sounds are not the typical musical expiratory (polyphonic) wheeze heard over the lung fields, or if there are unilateral signs, this should raise the suspicion of atypical causes of wheezing.
- The large majority of typical wheezy infants or preschool children do not require a great deal of investigation and in many cases a plain chest radiograph may be all that is needed.
- A history of failure to respond to anti-asthmatic medication is not particularly helpful in making the correct diagnosis in the wheezy infant or preschool child because:
     many typical wheezy infants do not respond to medications;
     the medication may not have been used for long enough;
     inhaled medications may not have been administered correctly;
     parents may be afraid of giving medications, especially corticosteroids.

EVALUATION OF SEVERITY OF WHEEZING ATTACKS

The first management decision for the typical infant or preschool child with recurrent wheezing attacks is to try to estimate the severity of the problem. The various guidelines for the management of asthma in adults and children are based upon steps of progressively increasing intensity, and contain suggestions for the evaluation of the severity of the problem in order to decide at which step to apply treatment.[1-3] In the older guidelines it was usually assumed that the patient was not receiving treatment when assessed or that the severity of the asthma could be determined by the treatment needed to achieve control – neither approach is particularly helpful. In the most recent modification of the Global Initiative for Asthma guidelines a much more realistic approach is adopted in which the treatment being taken modifies the assessment of severity based on symptoms.[4] However, even this more up-to-date approach only contains a grading system suitable for adults and there is no attempt to grade severity for the infant or preschool child. Asthma is classified as intermittent, mild persistent, moderate persistent or severe persistent based on clinical symptoms, physical activity and lung function, which are quite inappropriate for the very young wheezy child. Moreover, the grading system was designed for the typical asthmatic and it is unknown at present whether viral-induced wheezing behaves in the same way as asthma even in older children.

For the wheezy infant and preschool child it is far from certain that it is possible to grade the severity of the illness in the way it is graded in older children, let alone in adults, especially since it is necessary to rely heavily on the way the parents interpret the symptoms of their child. Any estimate of severity should be based on two major concerns:

- the amount of disturbance to the everyday life of the child and the family due to the wheezing or coughing attacks, including an estimate of the frequency of the attacks, their duration, whether the attacks are troublesome during the night and whether parents miss work to take care of the child;
- the severity of the attacks, including an estimate as to whether the attacks interfere with normal feeding and sleeping, and whether they require unscheduled visits to the doctor, emergency room or hospitalizations.

MANAGEMENT PLAN FOR THE WHEEZY INFANT AND PRESCHOOL CHILD

An alternative, and eminently simple approach, is to concentrate on the age and background of the child, the frequency of attacks and the response to a graded approach to treatment.

It is expected that there will be symptom-free intervals of weeks or months between attacks in the typical wheezy infant during which time treatment can be significantly reduced or stopped. The absence of symptom-free intervals, or the onset of attacks in an older infant, especially in the absence of an atopic background, is an indication to seek an atypical cause for the wheezing.

Some infants and children do not respond to treatment, which may be because they do not have asthma, it may be because infantile atopic wheezing or viral-induced wheezing is unresponsive, or it may be because they are not receiving their treatment properly. When a child is not responding to correctly administered medication in an appropriate dose, especially a corticosteroid, there is no reason for it to be continued and the treatment should be withdrawn to reduce the risk of harmful side effects.

A practical scheme based on these principles for the treatment of wheezing in the very young is given in Figure 7.1 and Table 7.1. The recommended steps for treatment on which the child should be placed are given in Figure 7.1 with more details of what these treatment steps entail being given in Table 7.1.

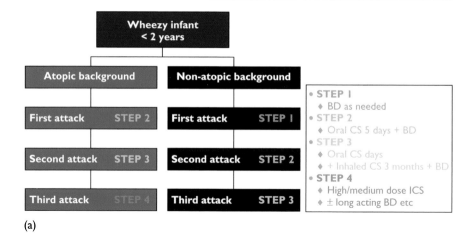

(a)

(b)

Figure 7.1

Treatment steps for recurrently wheezy infants (a) < 2 years of age and (b) between the ages of 2 and 6.

Determination of treatment steps for infants in the first two years of life
(Figure. 7.1a)

For infants in the first two years of life it is suggested that the treatment steps be related to the number of attacks and whether or not the infant has a personal or family background of atopy. After the first attack, subsequent attacks are treated with progressively more powerful medication, but if there is an atopic background the treatment is begun one step higher at each stage. The treatment of the wheezy infant is essentially a clinical trial and it cannot be expected that all will respond to medication, even to more powerful treatment with a corticosteroid.

Determination of treatment steps for preschool children between the ages of 2 and 6 (Figure 7.1b)

For preschool children between the ages of 2 and 6 the situation is more complicated and takes more account of the response to treatment.

Children with no previous attacks in the first two years of life having their first or second attack begin on step 2 (short course of oral corticosteroids), while those who have their third or subsequent attacks begin on step 3 (medium-term inhaled corticosteroids). If they respond well but relapse when the treatment is stopped, step 3 should be repeated, or extended for 6–12 months before stopping if they repeatedly relapse. Children who do not respond well to the first or subsequent courses of treatment at step 3 should move to step 4 (higher dose inhaled corticosteroid or supplementary treatment to low-dose corticosteroid). This should be continued for about 3–6 months, after which an attempt should be made to reduce treatment, especially the corticosteroid. If the child relapses at this time, step 4 will need to be resumed and attempts at reduction of treatment undertaken every few months. For those children who do not respond well to step 4 within 1–2 months, the actions outlined in step 5 should be considered. These include a search for atypical causes of wheezing which may have been missed and a 3–4 week course of oral corticosteroids in case the inhaled drug has not been taken regularly or adequately. If there is still no response, the corticosteroid treatment should be withdrawn since the infant is clearly deriving no benefit from this therapy.

For those children who have had previous attacks, the approach to stepwise treatment is similar. However, they should start on step 3 even if this was the first or second attack above the age of 2 years and on step 4 if this was the third or subsequent attack, since they would be classified as children who relapsed after stopping step 3 or who responded poorly to step 3. The move to step 5 should be determined as for the children with no attacks in the first two years of life.

Treatment steps for infants and preschool children (Table 7.1)

Step 1

For this step, treatment is given as needed until the attack is over, usually within 5–10 days, using an inhaled selective β_2-agonist bronchodilator and supplemental oxygen for those who are significantly hypoxic (saturation about < 92–93%). In acute viral bronchiolitis, epinephrine (adrenaline) by inhalation may be used instead.

Step 2

In this step, apart from giving an inhaled bronchodilator on an as-needed basis, the child is given a short course of a systemic corticosteroid such as prednisolone 1–2 mg/kg daily for 5 days.

Step 3

This step involves a short course of systemic corticosteroids (as in step 2) followed by medium-term treatment (about 3 months) of controller medication. Inhaled cortico-steroids are now widely accepted for this purpose and most would agree that a total daily dose of 200–400 µg is reasonable. Although it is traditional to give this in two divided doses, there are some data showing that for at least one corticosteroid a single daily dose can be used. In children with milder attacks, an alternative is a leukotriene receptor antagonist given by mouth, but the response varies, with some children responding well and others showing little or no response.

Step 4

In this step the intensity of treatment is increased either by doubling the daily dose of inhaled corticosteroid or by adding another regular medication to the same dose of

Table 7.1 Treatment steps with details of treatment	
Treatment step	Details of treatment
1	Treatment as needed until attack is over Reliever (bronchodilator), nebulized selective β_2-agonist preferred If RSV infection likely, alternative is nebulized epinephrine Oxygen if very distressed
2	Treatment as needed until attack is over Reliever (bronchodilator), nebulized selective β_2-agonist preferred Short-term oral corticosteroid for 5 days

3	Reliever (bronchodilator), nebulized selective β_2-agonist preferred
	Short-term oral corticosteroid for 5 days
	Controller (2–3 months):
	   low-dose inhaled corticosteroid or
	   trial of leukotriene antagonist in mild cases

4	Reliever (bronchodilator), nebulized selective β_2-agonist preferred
	Controller (long-term):
	   double-dose inhaled corticosteroid or
	   low-dose inhaled corticosteroid plus leukotriene antagonist or
	   long-acting inhaled β_2-agonist

5	Look for atypical causes of wheezing:
	   no atypical cause found – systemic corticosteroid for 3–4 weeks
	   no response to corticosteroid – withdraw controller treatment

RSV, Respiratory syncytial virus.

inhaled corticosteroid as in step 3. There are no data available to justify a particular steroid-sparing regimen in the very young child. By analogy with older children and adults, it is reasonable to try adding a regular daily dose of a long-acting selective β_2-agonist or a leukotriene receptor antagonist. While methyl xanthine derivatives were popular in the past, these agents tend to have side effects in the very young, especially hyperactivity, and are no longer recommended.

Step 5

The most important elements of step 5 are:

- to reconsider the possibility that the child has an atypical cause of wheezing and not one of the typical causes;
- that inhaled medications are not being administered efficiently;
- that the child is simply not responsive to any medication.

The differential diagnosis of wheezing in the infant and preschool child is considered fully in Chapter 6. There is always a real possibility with young children that inhaled medications are not being given correctly (see below) and therefore it is always worth trying a 3–4 week course of oral corticosteroid therapy before finally concluding that the child is not steroid responsive.

MEDICATIONS USED IN THE MANAGEMENT PLAN FOR THE WHEEZY INFANT AND PRESCHOOL CHILD

Relievers (bronchodilators)

Short-acting β_2-agonists

Short-acting relievers or bronchodilators give relatively rapid relief of symptoms and are believed to work predominantly by relaxation of airway smooth muscle (although several other effects on the airways may contribute to their anti-asthmatic effects). Relievers have no effect on the chronic inflammation of asthma and it is far from certain that they are effective in very young children,[10,15] although a minority of studies have shown an effect.[16] The most commonly used agents for wheezy infants are the short-acting β_2-agonists which, although they can be given by mouth, are normally given by inhalation as this appears to be more effective. In those infants who respond, the relief of symptoms should be almost immediate. Side effects can occur and include muscle tremor, tachycardia and even hypokalemia if used in excessive doses. Restlessness may be very troublesome in some infants.

Long-acting β_2-agonists

There is little or no experience with the clinical use of the long-acting bronchodilators in very young children and in many countries they are not yet licensed for use in in this age group. However, Primhak et al[17] undertook a dose-ranging study of salmeterol in infants of 8–45 months of age using the ability to reduce the response to a bronchial provocational challenge (PCwheeze). They found that a dose of 50–100 µg delivered through a spacer was effective. Since these drugs are accepted as being useful add-on steroid-sparing agents in older children, it seems reasonable to try them at step 4 in the wheezy infant and preschool guidelines described above, provided this is permitted by the local regulatory authorities.

Methyl xanthines

This group of compounds, including theophylline and its derivatives, are classified as bronchodilators, but relatively high doses are needed for airway smooth muscle relaxation. These drugs were very popular in some countries for treating asthma in children because they are given orally and slow-release preparations are available, making dosing simpler. Although they are quite effective in children with asthma there are only a few older studies of their use in the very young and in these the results were not particularly good.[18] Moreover, these agents are prone to cause side effects, especially in infants, including nausea, vomiting and restlessness, and cannot therefore be recommended for this age group.

Anticholinergic bronchodilators

This class of drugs inhibit cholinergic reflex bronchoconstriction and reduce vagal cholinergic tone. These agents have become quite popular for treating acute attacks of asthma in older children, especially in combination with a short-acting β_2-agonist.[19] Groggins et al[20] found that ipratropium was as effective as salbutamol in preschool children, but their value in the very young child has not been established.[21]

Controllers (anti-inflammatory agents)

The term controller implies treatments that suppress the underlying inflammatory process in asthmatic airways and in this sense prevent attacks developing in response to environmental triggers. Glucocorticoids are the only drugs that have been shown conclusively to significantly reduce the inflammation in asthmatic airways but other agents do have controller actions. Since it is by no means certain that the inflammation in viral-induced wheeze in infants is the same as that in atopic wheezing, nor that the inflammation in the atopic wheezy infant is the same as in the older asthmatic child, the actions of controller medications and indications for their use in the young child are somewhat speculative.

Corticosteroids

Inhaled corticosteroids are becoming the controllers of choice in the management of children with asthma. Their mode of action in reducing inflammation is complex and involves a number of mechanisms by which they affect metabolic pathways, concerning the manufacture and release of cytokines, mediators and expression of certain genes. In asthmatics, these agents reduce symptoms within days, improve lung function over days to weeks and reduce airway hyperresponsiveness over several months. There are a number of well-controlled studies showing that inhaled cortico-steroids can reduce symptoms in wheezy infants and preschool children, although no distinction has usually been made between atopic and non-atopic children who are all considered to be asthmatics by the authors of these studies. In the study of de Blic et al,[22] children between the ages of 1.6 and 4.9 were given an inhaled corticosteroid or placebo for 12 weeks. There were fewer exacerbations in the treated children than in the placebo group, even though more of the placebo group had a parent with atopic disease. Similar studies lasting 8–12 weeks in children between the ages of 2.1 and 5.8[23] and 1.0 and 3.9,[24] of whom the majority had a personal or family background of atopy, showed an improvement in symptoms, which was dose related in one of the studies. A small improvement of bronchial responsivity to cold-air inhalation but not to methacholine was found in one study.[23] Some studies have been undertaken to determine whether or not the short-term administration of corticosteroids can alter the course of a wheezing attack apparently induced by a viral infection, although in none of these studies was the viral origin proved nor was the atopic status of the children defined. In these studies of children between 6 months and 5 years of age, there was a reduction of symptoms in the short term compared with attacks treated by placebo.[25–27] However, a Cochrane Library study concluded that, while episodic high-dose inhaled corticosteroids were partially effective in mild episodic apparently viral-induced wheeze in children, including the very young, there was no evidence that low-dose maintenance therapy was helpful in preventing viral-induced attacks of wheeze.[28]

In adults it is generally believed that the dose–response curve of corticosteroids is rel-atively flat with little extra benefit being obtained from the use of large doses. This has not been established for infants and young children and there are studies which clearly show a beneficial dose–response effect in wheezy preschool children.[24] These studies explored the use of fluticasone propionate in doses up to 200 μcg daily, delivered from a pressurized metered dose inhaler through a low-volume spacer-holding chamber. A major difficulty in giving inhaled corticosteroids to very young children concerns the method of administration and this may account for some of the dose effect, since more of the larger dose is likely to reach the lungs. However, these drugs are also systemically active and 400 μcg daily of either fluticasone propionate or budesonide has been shown to have a small slowing effect on lower leg growth.[29] Again, poor inhalation technique might result in more systemic absorption of the drug. Careful consideration should be given to using higher doses for infants and preschool children who do not respond. Alternatively, steroid-sparing strategies such as combining a lower dose of cortico-steroid with a leukotriene antagonist or long-acting β₂-agonist should be tried.

The issue of the possible side effects from inhaled corticosteroids is, of course, very important, especially in children. Local side effects are less common in children than in adults but there are reports of systemic side effects on growth and adrenal function after inhaled steroids.[30–32] However, clinically evident adrenal insufficiency has not been a problem in children taking reasonable doses of inhaled corticosteroids provided they have not also been receiving oral corticosteroids. Wolthers and Pedersen[33] have demonstrated that even normal doses of inhaled corticosteroids can reduce lower leg growth measured by knemometry in a dose-dependent fashion in the short term. On the other hand, in a long-term study of asthmatic children, Ninan and Russell[34] showed that inadequate control of asthma and not the use of corticosteroids adversely affected growth. A meta-analysis of the effect of oral and inhaled corticosteroids on growth in 810 children found a small degree of growth impairment with oral therapy but none with inhaled therapy, even with higher doses, longer use or, worse, asthma.[35] Final adult height has also been shown to be normal in children treated with inhaled corticosteroids.[36,37] It should be remembered that poorly controlled asthma can retard growth.

As with older children, short-term systemic effects of inhaled corticosteroids have been found by knemometry in 1–3-year-old children treated for 4 weeks with inhaled corticosteroids,[29] but this does not seem to have any long-term adverse effects. Reid et al[38] followed 40 children between the ages of 0.33 and 2.8 (mean 1.4 years of age) with what they termed 'severe asthma' for 6 months to 1.5 years while they received between 1000 and 2000 µg daily of nebulized budesonide. They found no evidence of any adverse effect on growth in these infants and young children.

Oral corticosteroids are not normally used for regular daily treatment of asthmatic children on a long-term basis but they are indicated for short courses aimed at terminating an attack as rapidly as possible. Some infants and young children are quite unwilling to accept any form of inhaled corticosteroid therapy and for these children consideration should be given to using an oral corticosteroid. For those children who are not controlled, despite apparently receiving adequate inhaled corticosteroids, there is always the possibility that they are not being taken properly, so before withdrawing corticosteroids a 3–4 week trial of oral therapy should be considered. In these situations it is preferable to give the oral preparation as a single dose every other morning since, at least in older children, this has long been accepted as being far less likely to have systemic side effects.[30,39] The side effects of prolonged daily oral steroid therapy (> 1–2 months) or frequent short courses (more than once every 1–2 months for several months) include all the usual systemic effects and an adverse effect on growth.

Leukotriene receptor antagonists

These are a relatively new class of drug for the control of asthma and are now available for children as young as two years of age, which makes them of potential value for the wheezy preschool child. Their great advantage is that they are active orally but their true role in management has not yet been fully established, although they are mentioned in the Global Initiative for Asthma guidelines[4] for use in moderate persistent asthma in children. In a multicenter study of children between the ages of 2 and 5, montelukast, administered for 12 weeks as a 4 mg chewable tablet, produced significant improvements compared with placebo in multiple parameters of asthma control.[40] However, the differences from the control group, although significant, were very small and the children were in any case quite mildly affected as judged by their baseline symptoms. In a related study it was shown that montelukast could protect these young children against cold-air-induced asthma,[41] which suggests that leukotrienes may play a role even in the very young wheezy child. It has become apparent that the response to these agents at all ages varies widely and unpredictably from patient to patient, with some responding well and some not at all.

Cromones

These drugs, which include sodium cromoglycate and nedocromil sodium, were popular in the past as controller medications for children with mild to moderate persistent asthma in whom they were shown to be effective over the short and long term.[42] These agents act through mast cell stabilization, inhibition of sensory nerve activation and inhibitory effects on several types of inflammatory cell. Cromolyn sodium is almost totally without any adverse effects but is only effective by inhalation and is relatively short acting, requiring the child to take three to four doses a day. In the preschool child, sodium cromoglycate has not been convincingly shown to be effective. Some earlier studies suggested that it was helpful;[43] however, a large recent double-blind parallel group study of 167 children between the ages of 1 and 4 for 5 months found no clinical differences in outcome, and it was suggested that the drug be dropped from the guidelines.[44]

DELIVERY DEVICES FOR INHALATION SUITABLE FOR INFANTS AND YOUNG CHILDREN

A major factor in the management of wheezy infants and preschool children is the ability or otherwise of the child to take medications, especially inhaled medications, and the ability of the parents to administer them. It is quite useless to prescribe a metered dose inhaler without a spacer for most young children and quite unrealistic to expect parents to administer medications through a nebulizer to a screaming infant who is terrified by the noise of the compressor. The choice of inhalation device must be tailored to each child and its efficient use ensured by education of the child and family (and sometimes even the doctor). The most commonly used inhalation devices are the pressurized metered dose inhaler with some type of spacer-holding chamber (pMDI-SP) and the jet nebulizer (NEB), but many children > 4 years of age can also use dry powder inhalers (DPI) successfully.[45] The ultrasonic nebulizer is used much less often for the delivery of asthma medications.

Pressurized metered dose inhaler with spacer (pMDI-SP)

Because many patients, both young and old, are unable to coordinate well enough to use an pMDI correctly, various holding chambers (spacers) have been developed which are placed between the pMDI and the patient. The drug is inhaled from the chamber and coordination with the firing of the pMDI is no longer important. Most spacers have some type of non-rebreathing valve. The pMDI to be used with the spacer should be shaken immediately before use and fixed upright in the appropriate aperture in the spacer. Most infants and younger children will use a face-mask attachment with the spacer and it is essential for the parents to ensure that the mask fits closely to the face and that there is no leak around it, which would completely invalidate its use. The child should continue to breathe normally without pause from the spacer while the pMDI is fired. About 5–6 breaths are usually sufficient to inspire the contents of the spacer and there is no need to continue longer provided the mask is well sealed to the face. The parents should try to observe the movement of the valves in spacers for infants to ensure that they are functioning and that there is no leak around the mask. When the treatment calls for two or more doses of medication, it is important that each dose be taken separately and it is not recommended that the spacer be loaded with several doses. When using a pMDI-SP with a face mask to administer corticosteroids to an infant or young child it is recommended that the face be washed afterwards to reduce exposure of the skin around the mouth to the drug. Always remember that some infants and young children are terrified of face masks and spacers, and the parents may find it totally impossible to administer medication to their infant with this type of device. The advantages of the pMDI-SP inhaler combination include the following:

- coordination unimportant;
- can be used by patients of all ages;
- may reduce systemic absorption of corticosteroids;
- relatively inexpensive.

The disadvantages of the pMDI-SP inhalers include the following:

- devices are somewhat bulky and inconvenient;
- valves sometimes stick or become incompetent;
- some infants struggle against the mask and a good seal may not be obtained.

Jet nebulizer (NEB)

The oldest types of inhalation devices delivered the drug by using a hand pump or even a pressure steam kettle to nebulize a solution and produce a cloud of medication which was inhaled. In its modern form this is accomplished by passing a jet of air from a compressor over a solution of the drug contained in a reservoir. The nebulizer should be set up according to the manufacturer's instructions and the appropriate amount of drug, diluted with saline if necessary, should be placed in the reservoir. Most NEB reservoirs must be held in a vertical position so that the drug does not spill over into the exit from the nebulization chamber. This can easily occur if the device is used for a child who is asleep in bed. The patient should breathe normally from the face mask while the compressor is run continuously until a cloud of drug is no longer apparent at the exit of the device – normally 5–6 minutes is long enough. If for some reason the child stops using the NEB, it should be turned off until inhalation is resumed. Some infants and young children are terrified by nebulizers because of the noise made by the compressor. The advantages of the NEB inhalers include the following:

- coordination unimportant;
- can be used for all ages.

The disadvantages of the NEB inhalers include the following:

- cumbersome equipment;
- requires a source of electricity;

- expensive;
- noisy;
- treatment takes a long time;
- disliked by some infants, loathed by others.

Remember, some infants and young children are unwilling to accept metered dose inhalers and spacers, some are unwilling to accept nebulizers, and some are unwilling to accept either. It is absolutely essential for the pediatrician to observe the manner in which the parents administer the medication to their child through the device and if it appears unlikely that this can be done effectively, an alternative method of treatment should be considered.

Dry powder inhaler (DPI)

For many years devices have been available for the delivery of dry powders of medications diluted with suitable inert compounds. These do not contain propellants and are only activated by the inspiratory effort of the patient. There are several different types of DPI and it is important to follow the instructions for priming the device as recommended by the manufacturer. Spacers or face masks are not available for use with DPI and the child must be able to breathe out before closing the lips firmly around the mouthpiece and then inspire rapidly and deeply. Children > 4–5 years of age can learn to use DPI,[45] which are much more convenient than either pMDI-SP or NEB devices. When taking corticosteroids from a DPI it is recommended that the mouth be washed out afterwards to reduce buccal absorption of the drug. The advantages of DPI inhalers include the following:

- coordination unimportant;
- can be used for children from about 4–5 years of age;
- devices are small and portable.

The disadvantages of DPI inhalers include the following:

- require rapid inspiration;
- not suitable for children < 4 years of age;
- relatively expensive.

TREATING THE WHEEZY INFANT OR PRESCHOOL CHILD WHO DOES NOT RESPOND TO MEDICATION

There is no doubt that a large number of wheezy infants and preschool children are not responsive to medications which are effective in childhood asthma. Even some atopic wheezy infants and preschool children do not respond to anti-asthmatic medications.[10] The management of these children, whose wheezing is probably viral induced, is problematic and there is no general consensus.

Parents expect their pediatrician to provide treatment for their symptomatic child but at the start of treatment there is no reliable way of knowing whether or not the child will respond to medication. For this reason, a trial of therapy should be attempted as described earlier, which usually includes an oral corticosteroid together with a bronchodilator on a short-term basis. If there is no response, and it is certain that the child is receiving the medication regularly and in an effective manner, it is not worth persisting with the corticosteroid. However, it is almost impossible to be sure that the infant or preschool child is really receiving an inhaled corticosteroid regularly and effectively, and hence, as suggested earlier, a short trial of oral therapy may be indicated. Other controller medications such a leukotriene antagonists or sodium cromoglycate are unlikely to help in this type of infant. Having decided that the usual type of controller medications are not indicated, the use of an inhaled bronchodilator on an as-needed basis is almost irresistible, which at best may provide a little relief and at worse is not harmful or likely to cause side effects.

Unfortunately, many of these infants and young children continue to receive corticosteroids, even though they are receiving no benefit from the medication, and this, of course, is undesirable.

When faced with the parents of a young child who is not steroid responsive, the best plan is to explain to the parents the nature of the problem, that anti-asthma medication is not indicated in their child, that the unwarranted use of corticosteroids can be harmful and that the situation is likely to improve with time.

If the child is indeed a young potential asthmatic who is not responsive it is very likely that over the next few months the child will begin to respond to regular anti-asthmatic medication. If the wheezing follows RSV bronchiolitis it is very likely to become less severe over the next few months and the very large majority of such infants do not continue to wheeze into later childhood. The exact position of infants or preschool children with other types of viral-induced wheeze is uncertain at this time.

For those non-responsive infants or preschool children with wheezing that continues to be troublesome, it is reasonable to undertake a trial of anti-asthmatic medication from time to time to determine whether or not they have become responsive.

In infants or preschool children with troublesome and persistent symptoms who do not respond to medication which is being given in effective manner, consideration should always be given to the other diagnoses as described in Chapter 6. The child should be referred to a specialist in pediatric respiratory disease if:

- there is doubt about diagnosis or suspicion of atypical wheezing;
- there is failure to thrive;
- the child responds only to high-dose inhaled corticosteroids;
- the child requires treatment with oral corticosteroids;
- the child or the parents have compliance or psychological problems.

EFFECT OF TREATMENT ON LONG-TERM PROGNOSIS

While it is now commonly recommended that treatment with inhaled corticosteroids should be started early in asthma, there appear to be very few objective studies to substantiate this policy. More controlled prospective studies are needed in children to determine the validity of the clinical impression that the prognosis of childhood asthma has improved with the earlier use of inhaled corticosteroids. Prospective studies have investigated the effect of corticosteroid treatment during the acute phase of bronchiolitis in infancy on subsequent wheezing during early childhood. Thus, van Woensel et al[46] performed a controlled prospective follow-up study after a randomized double-blind placebo-controlled intervention with oral prednisolone in the acute phase of bronchiolitis in 54 infants < 2 years of age hospitalized for RSV bronchiolitis. At a mean of 5 years of age, 47 patients had completed their follow-up. They found no significant differences between the prednisolone- and the placebo-treated group in the number of patients with transient wheezing (8 versus 17%), persistent wheezing (42 versus 31%) or late-onset wheezing (17 versus 13%). Reijonen et al[47] looked at the effect of both an inhaled corticosteroid and cromolyn sodium as anti-inflammatory treatment during the acute phase on the prognosis after 3 years of bronchiolitic infants. The anti-inflammatory therapy was given for 16 weeks; 29 patients received cromolyn sodium, 31 patients received budesonide and 29 control patients received no therapy. Fourteen (48%) patients in the former cromolyn group, 15 (48%) in the former budesonide group, and 16 (55%) in the control group had current asthma. They concluded that anti-inflammatory therapy for 4 months had no influence on the occurrence of asthma 3 years after wheezing in infancy.

In older children with established asthma, Agertoft and Pedersen[48] looked at the effect of the delay in starting corticosteroid therapy on prognosis. They followed 216 children of 6.2 years of age at the start with mild to moderate asthma for 1–2 years without steroids and then for 3–6 years while being treated with inhaled budesonide and compared them with a control group that continued without budesonide. Although this was not a properly randomized study it appears that treatment with the corticosteroid significantly reduced the number of hospitalizations compared with the run-in period and controls. They noted that the earlier the onset of corticosteroid therapy after onset of asthma, the greater the improvement in the forced expiratory volume in 1 second (FEV_1). In a later study, the same authors followed children between the ages of 5 and 12 with mild to moderate asthma taking either budesonide, nedocromil or placebo for 4–6 years.[37] There was no significant difference between treatments and placebo in the primary outcome, i.e. the degree of change in FEV_1. In the Childhood Asthma Management Program (CAMP) research group study, 1041 children between the ages of 5 and 12 with mild to moderate asthma were randomly assigned to receive 200 μcg of inhaled corticosteroid (budesonide) or 8 mg of nedocromil or placebo twice daily for 4–6 years.[49] There was no significant difference between treatments and placebo in the primary outcome, i.e. the degree of change in FEV_1, expressed as a percentage of the predicted value after the administration of a bronchodilator. As compared with the children assigned to placebo, the children assigned to receive budesonide improved in terms of several clinical markers, while nedocromil significantly reduced urgent care visits and courses of prednisone. The mean increase in height in the budesonide group was 1.1 cm less than in the placebo group but this difference was evident mostly within the first year. The height increase was similar in the nedocromil and placebo groups. The conclusions of this study were that in children with mild to moderate asthma, neither budesonide nor nedocromil is better than placebo in terms of lung function, but inhaled budesonide improves airway responsiveness and provides better control of asthma than placebo or nedocromil. The side effects of budesonide were limited to a small, transient reduction in growth velocity. To what extent these observations in older, established asthmatics can be applied to wheezy infants and preschool children is uncertain, especially because the attacks are much more likely to be intermittent rather than continuous in the younger age group.

For those older infants and preschool children who develop fairly continuous symptoms, and who clearly respond to controller medication so that they have the characteristics of older children with asthma, it would seem reasonable to continue treatment until the child, hopefully, grows out of the condition. For those who do not respond, there can be little if any justification in persisting with medications such as corticosteroids which can produce potentially harmful effects in some children.

REFERENCES

1. National Institutes of Health (NIH). *Expert Panel Report 2. Guidelines for the diagnosis and management of asthma.* NIH Publication No. 97–4051. (NIH, National Heart, Lung, and Blood Institute: Bethesda, MD, 1997.)

2. The British Thoracic Society and others. The British guidelines on asthma management 1995 review and position statement. *Thorax* 1997; **52 (Suppl 1)**: S1–S21.

3. Pediatric Asthma Promoting Best Practice. Guide for Managing Asthma in Children. (American Academy of Allergy, Asthma and Immunology. Rochester, New York, 1999.)

4. Global Initiative for Asthma. *Global strategy for asthma management and prevention.* (National Institutes of Health: Bethesda, MD, 2002.)

5. Martinez FD, Morgan WJ, Wright AL et al and the Group Health Medical Associates' Personnel. Diminished lung function as a predisposing factor for wheezing respiratory illness in infants. *N Engl J Med* 1988; **319**: 1112–17.

6. Dabbous IA, Tkachyk JS, Stamm SJ. A double blind study on the effect of corticosteroids in the treatment of bronchiolitis. *Pediatrics* 1966; **37**: 477–84.

7. Yaffe SJ, Weiss CF, Cann HM et al. Should steroids be used in treating bronchiolitis? *Pediatrics* 1970; **46**: 640–2.

8. Kimpen JL, Schaad UB. Treatment of respiratory syncytial virus bronchiolitis: 1995 poll of members of the European Society for Paediatric Infectious Diseases. *Pediatr Infect Dis J* 1997; **16**: 479–81.

9. Phelan P, Williams HE. Sympathomimetic drugs in acute viral bronchiolitis. Their effect on pulmonary resistance. *Pediatrics* 1969; **44**: 493–7.

10. Lenney W, Milner AD. At what age do bronchodilator drugs work. *Arch Dis Child* 1978; **53**: 532–5.

11. Bertrand P, Aranibar H, Castro E, Sanchez I. Efficacy of nebulized epinephrine versus salbutamol in hospitalized infants with bronchiolitis. *Pediatr Pulmonol* 2001; **31**: 284–8.

12. Stokes GM, Milner AD, Hodges IGC et al. Nebulised therapy in acute bronchiolitis in infancy. *Arch Dis Child* 1983; **58**: 279–83.

13. Lodrup Carlsen KC, Carlsen KH. Inhaled nebulized adrenaline improves lung function in infants with acute bronchiolitis. *Resp Med* 2000; **94**: 709–14.

14. Numa AH, Williams GD, Dakin CJ. The effect of nebulized epinephrine on respiratory mechanics and gas exchange in bronchiolitis. *Am J Resp Crit Care Med* 2001; **164**: 86–91.

15. Hayden MJ, Wildhaber JH, LeSouef PN. Bronchodilator responsiveness testing using raised volume forced expiration in recurrently wheezing infants. *Pediatr Pulmonol* 1998; **26**: 35–41.

16. Kraemer R, Frey U, Sommer CW, Russi E. Short-term effect of albuterol, delivered via a new auxillary device, in wheezy

infants. *Am Rev Resp Dis* 1991; **144**: 347–51.

17. Primhak RA, Smith CM, Yong SC et al. The bronchoprotective effect of inhaled salmeterol in preschool children: a dose-ranging study. *Eur Resp J* 1999; **13**: 78–81.

18. Loftus BG, Price JF. Treatment of asthma in preschool children with slow release theophylline. *Arch Dis Child* 1985; **60**: 770–2.

19. Schuh S, Johnson DW, Callahan S et al. Efficacy of frequent nebulized ipratropium bromide added to frequent high-dose albuterol therapy in severe childhood asthma. *J Pediatr* 1995; **126**: 639–45.

20. Groggins RC, Milner AD, Stokes GM. Bronchodilator effects of clemastine, ipratropium bromide, and salbutamol in preschool children with asthma. *Arch Dis Child* 1981; **56**: 342–4.

21. Everard ML, Bara A, Kurian M et al. Anticholinergic drugs for wheeze in children under the age of two years. (Cochrane Review). In: The Cochrane Library, Issue 2, 2002. Oxford: Update Software.

22. de Blic J, Delacourt C, Le Bourgeois M et al. Efficacy of nebulized budesonide in treatment of severe infantile asthma: a double-blind study. *J Allergy Clin Immunol* 1996; **98**: 14–20.

23. Nielsen KG, Bisgaard H. The effect of inhaled budesonide on symptoms, lung function, and cold air and methacholine responsiveness in 2- to 5-year-old asthmatic children. *Am J Resp Crit Care Med* 2000; **162**: 1500–6.

24. Bisgaard H, Gillies J, Groenewald M, Maden C. The effect of inhaled fluticasone propionate in the treatment of young asthmatic children: a dose comparison study. *Am J Resp Crit Care Med* 1999; **160**: 126–31.

25. Wilson NM, Silverman M. Treatment of acute, episodic asthma in preschool children using intermittent high dose inhaled steroids at home. *Arch Dis Child* 1990; **65**: 407–10.

26. Connett G, Lenney W. Prevention of viral induced asthma attacks using inhaled

budesonide. *Arch Dis Child* 1993; **68**: 85–7.

27. Svedmyr J, Nyberg E, Thunqvist P et al. Prophylactic intermittent treatment with inhaled corticosteroids of asthma exacerbations due to airway infections in toddlers. *Acta Paediatr* 1999; **88**: 42–7.

28. McKean M, Ducharme F. Inhaled steroids for episodic viral wheeze of childhood. (Cochrane Review). In: The Cochrane Library, Issue 1, 2002. Oxford: Update Software.

29. Anhoj J, Bisgaard AM, Bisgaard H. Systemic activity of inhaled steroids in 1- to 3-year-old children with asthma. *Pediatrics* 2002; **109**: E40–E43.

30. Nassif E, Weinberger M, Sherman B, Brown K. Extrapulmonary effects of maintenance corticoid therapy with alternate-day prednisone and inhaled beclomethasone in children with chronic asthma. *J Allergy Clin Immunol* 1987; **80**: 518–29.

31. Law CM, Marchant JL, Honour JW et al. Nocturnal adrenal suppression in asthmatic children taking inhaled beclomethasone dipropionate. *Lancet* 1986; **1**: 942–4.

32. Phillip M, Aviram M, Leiberman E et al. Integrated plasma cortisol concentration in children with asthma receiving long-term inhaled corticosteroids. *Pediatr Pulmonol* 1992; **12**: 84–9.

33. Wolthers OD, Pedersen S. Growth of asthmatic children during treatment with budesonide: a double blind trial. *Br Med J* 1991; **303**: 163–5.

34. Ninan TK, Russell G. Asthma, inhaled corticosteroid treatment and growth. *Arch Dis Child* 1992; **67**: 703–5.

35. Allen DB, Mullen M, Mullen B. A meta-analysis of the effect of oral and inhaled corticosteroids on growth. *J Allergy Clin Immunol* 1994; **93**: 967–76.

36. Balfour-Lynn L. Growth and childhood asthma. *Arch Dis Child* 1986; **61**: 1049–55.

37. Agertoft L, Pedersen S. Effect of long-term treatment with inhaled budesonide on adult height in children with asthma. *N Engl J Med* 2000; **343**: 1064–9.

38. Reid A, Murphy C, Steen HJ et al. Linear growth of very young asthmatic children treated with high-dose nebulized budesonide. *Acta Paediatr Scand* 1996; **85**: 421–4.

39. Falliers CJ, Chai H, Molk L et al. Pulmonary and adrenal effects of alternate day corticosteroid therapy. *J Allergy Clin Immunol* 1972; **49**: 156–66.

40. Knorr B, Franchi LM, Bisgaard H et al. Montelukast, a leukotriene receptor antagonist, for the treatment of persistent asthma in children aged 2 to 5 years. *Pediatrics* 2001; **108**: E48.

41. Bisgaard H, Nielsen KG. Bronchoprotection with a leukotriene receptor antagonist in asthmatic preschool children. *Am J Resp Crit Care Med* 2000; **162**: 187–90.

42. Silverman M, Connolly NM, Balfour-Lynn L, Godfrey S. Long-term trial of disodium cromoglycate and isoprenaline in children with asthma. *Br Med J* 1972; **3**: 378–81.

43. Cogswell JJ, Simpkiss MJ. Nebulised sodium cromoglycate in recurrently wheezy preschool children. *Arch Dis Child* 1985; **60**: 736–8.

44. Tasche MJA, van der Wouden JC, Uijen JHJM et al. Randomised placebo controlled trial of inhaled sodium cromoglycate in 1–4 year old children with moderate asthma. *Lancet* 1997; **360**: 1060–4.

45. Goren A, Noviski N, Avital A et al. Assessment of the ability of young children to use a powder inhaler device (Turbuhaler). *Pediatr Pulmonol* 1994; **18**: 77–80.

46. van Woensel JB, Kimpen JL, Sprikkelman AB et al. Long-term effects of prednisolone in the acute phase of bronchiolitis caused by respiratory syncytial virus. *Pediatr Pulmonol* 2000; **30**: 92–6.

47. Reijonen TM, Kotaniemi-Syrjanen A, Korhonen K, Korppi M. Predictors of asthma three years after hospital admission for wheezing in infancy. *Pediatrics* 2000; **106**: 1406–12.

48. Agertoft L, Pedersen S. Effects of long term treatment with an inhaled corticosteroid on growth and pulmonary function in asthmatic children. *Resp Med* 1994; **88**: 373–81.

49. The Childhood Asthma Management Program Research Group. Long-term effects of budesonide or nedocromil in children with asthma. *N Engl J Med* 2000; **343**: 1054–63.

8
Proposals for the future

INTRODUCTION

Two constant themes have recurred throughout this book. On the one hand, we have outlined the importance of events occurring during the first years of life as predictors and harbingers of the subsequent development of chronic respiratory symptoms and chronic obstructive disease later in life. On the other hand, we have stressed the lack of real, hard facts about the etiology and pathophysiology of the disease process occurring in the typical wheezy infant and preschool child, and the optimum approach to diagnosis and management. It is very difficult to explain why a condition that seems to be such an important risk factor for the development for subsequent chronic illnesses and that, at the same time, has such a strong impact in terms of morbidity during the first years of life has not, until recently, become the focus of interest of significant research and attention by the academic and business communities. It could be argued that there are significant limitations to our capacity to study any condition in infants and very young children. Regulatory institutions may also have contributed to making some of the most frequent illnesses affecting young children almost comparable (in terms of research interest) to the so-called 'orphan diseases', which are several orders of magnitude rarer and have only a tiny fraction of the impact that wheezing has on public health. Indeed, in most countries, regulatory agencies do not require that medicines that have been shown to be effective in the treatment of conditions that are clinically similar to early childhood wheezing are specifically tested in this age group. This has resulted in the bewildering situation described in Chapter 7 dealing with treatment of wheezing: most pediatricians and caregivers who treat children with wheezing know that medicines used to treat asthma in adults are much less effective in this age group, but are constrained to continue using them simply because there are few drugs that have been tested specifically in infants and young children. As physicians who have dedicated a significant part of our lives to the study, prevention and treatment of wheezing disorders in young children, we believe this situation is unacceptable and needs to be remedied.

While there have been important advances in our understanding of early childhood wheezing over recent years, there are still very large gaps in our knowledge and properly planned and well-executed studies are required. In this chapter, we shall attempt to point out where there is need for more research and how this might be approached, given the limitations imposed by the study of disease affecting very young children. We do not intend to consider research into the problem of the atypical wheezy infant or preschool child, as these relate to the specific individual diseases beyond the scope of this book. In our view there is need for research in five major fields.

STUDIES TO ESTABLISH THE RELATIONSHIP BETWEEN GENETIC PREDISPOSITION, ENVIRONMENTAL EXPOSURE, AND THE VARIOUS TYPES OF TYPICAL WHEEZING IN INFANCY AND EARLY CHILDHOOD

During the past 20 years, several studies have been started in which relatively large numbers of children were enrolled at birth and followed prospectively to determine the incidence of and risk factors for wheezing illnesses during the first years of life. All these studies have contributed significant new information, which is summarized elsewhere in this book. Perhaps one of the most important conclusions that can be reached from these studies is that although these different forms of wheezing are not easily distinguishable from a clinical point of view, it is crucial to develop tools to allow the clinician and the researcher to identify more accurately these different forms, and thus to develop strategies for prevention and treatment that would be specific for each of them. In order for such an effort to be successful, however, sufficiently large samples of children from different countries, ethnic backgrounds and socioeconomic conditions would need to be enrolled. Although efforts have been made in the past to concentrate enrollment on high-risk children, we believe that results of such studies could be misinterpreted and the conclusions reached from them applied to all young children with wheezing illnesses. We favor an approach where these longitudinal studies would enroll children selected randomly from the general population as newborns (or even earlier).

In addition, concomitant assessment will need to be made of environmental exposures and genetic variations known or suspected to be related to such exposures, and that are known or are suspected to influence the development of wheezing illnesses during the first years of life. Recent advances in the genomic revolution have allowed us to screen for a very large number of genetic variations present in the human genome and to do so in very large population samples. Moreover, it is very possible that, in the near future, technologies will become available that will allow for anonymous screening of the whole genome for potential association between marker polymorphisms and diseases of interest, in this case, wheezing disorders of infants and young children. These technologies will obviate the need to specifically define candidate genes and will allow the geneticist to simply determine if evidence for association exists in any gene anywhere in the genome with respect to such diseases of interest. Naturally, the best context in which to do such studies is one in which relevant environmental exposures have also been assessed. This seems to be a necessary step, because most genetic studies of asthma are demonstrating that the effects of any genetic variant on the disease is rather small and perhaps restricted to specific groups of individuals who have been exposed to certain environmental factors that interact, directly or indirectly, with such variants. There is no reason to believe that wheezing illnesses of the early years will show a different genetic pattern. The promise of such studies is to be able to predict which children who are exposed to certain environmental factors are at the highest risk of developing wheezing and, therefore, to center attention, both in terms of prevention and treatment, on these children.

An additional advantage of these types of studies would be that they would be able to establish the true incidence of the various types of wheezing in infancy and early childhood at different ages and in different communities. At the same time, these studies could be the basis for longer term assessment of the prognosis in later childhood and adult life of the various types of wheezing that occur in infancy and early childhood.

One drawback of prospective studies is their considerable expense and difficulty. They often require very large numbers of subjects and particular attention needs to be paid to minimizing losses to follow-up. They also place considerable burden on the study participants. In addition, it may not be easy to keep track of children belonging to populations of special interest from the point of view of wheezing in early life, e.g. those of lower socioeconomic status or belonging to certain ethnic groups. Moreover, studies will be difficult to conduct in underdeveloped countries, who suffer a considerable part of the burden for these diseases, due to the lack of resources and the almost complete absence of well-trained researchers with sufficient time to pursue such studies. However, we are convinced that the results obtained from the currently available longitudinal studies more than outweigh their costs and more than justify the efforts needed to conduct them. These studies have very significantly changed the way we understand childhood obstructive respiratory diseases and have opened new and important areas for research. Future studies carry with them the promise of similar influences on our current paradigms.

STUDIES OF THE GENETICS, RISK FACTORS FOR AND THE TREATMENT OF ACUTE BRONCHIOLITIS DUE TO RESPIRATORY SYNCYTIAL VIRUS (RSV)

Although acute bronchiolitis can be considered one of the clinical expressions of wheezing in early childhood, we dedicated a separate chapter to this matter because of the many issues that are specific to acute RSV infection in early life. This being one of the main causes of morbidity of any type in this age group, a specific approach towards a better understanding of the epidemiologic and genetic factors that are associated with acute RSV infection is very necessary. By this same token, we consider that there is an extremely high priority for the development of specific treatments to be used during acute episodes of RSV bronchiolitis and, at the same time, for the development of a vaccine for RSV. With respect to the first point, we have made clear in Chapter 2 about RSV illness that there is no specific anti-RSV treatment currently available that is widely used in major academic and clinical centers. Although ribavirin is approved for use during acute bronchiolitis in many countries, its effectiveness is under question and many clinicians believe that it does not play a role in most cases of acute bronchiolitis. It is possible that the use of an anti-viral agent at a time when the lower respiratory illness is already in full clinical expression may not be appropriate, because most of the effects may be associated with the immune response to the virus and its invasive properties, which cannot be controlled by such agents administered at such a late phase of the illness. Perhaps better methods for early screening of RSV in infants who will go on to develop bronchiolitis would allow the administration of such anti-viral drugs at an earlier stage of the disease.

There is little doubt that the availability of passive immunization approaches to the prevention of RSV illness has significantly decreased the morbidity of RSV illness in children at very high risk of severe disease. However, these treatments cannot be used on a large scale because they are either cumbersome to administer or very expensive.

In the future, treatments for the acute illness may come from a better understanding of the immune mechanisms associated with acute RSV bronchiolitis. A lot has been learned about these mechanisms in animal models of acute RSV, but unfortunately these models are artificial and are obtained using animals that do not develop spontaneous RSV disease in nature. There is no doubt that increased knowledge about RSV disease in humans is hampered by justified concerns about potential harmful effects of the invasive techniques that may be needed to understand these mechanisms in the lung. This will be discussed further below.

Finally, the lack of a vaccine or active immunization for RSV constitutes, in our opinion, a major weakness in today's fight against respiratory illness worldwide. It is clear that the unwanted side effects and even deaths that occurred during trials with formalin-inactivated RSV vaccines 30 years ago have justifiably made researchers involved in this field very cautious in trying any new vaccines in humans. However, we are convinced that if more resources were dedicated to RSV, and if infants who develop severe RSV illness or who die as a consequence of these illnesses had a strong and dedicated advocacy group such as, for example, patients with HIV do, major advances would also be made in this field.

STUDIES OF THE IMMUNOLOGIC BASIS OF WHEEZING DISEASES OF INFANCY AND EARLY CHILDHOOD

In this book we have pointed out how limited our knowledge is about the immunologic basis of typical wheezing illnesses in infancy and early childhood. The scanty information available, both from samples obtained from blood and from lung and airway tissue, clearly supports the contention that the immune mechanisms involved in wheezing illnesses in this age group are different from those known to be associated with asthma and other wheezing syndromes later in life. As we have also pointed out, it appears that at least certain forms of recurrent wheezing in infancy and early childhood are associated with a progressive increase in bronchial responsiveness and a progressive deterioration of lung function. The immune mechanisms that determine these changes are not understood. We believe that this is a significant hiatus in our knowledge, which hampers the development of strategies for the primary and secondary prevention of asthma, especially in individuals known to be at high risk for this disease due to their familial background.

We are aware that the ethical approaches towards studies involving human subjects are changing very dramatically in Western societies. We also understand that the issues involved are highly complex, concerning the right of society to include unaware and often unwilling children in studies that may be associated with discomfort and increased risk (albeit minimal) of undesirable consequences. We wholeheartedly support the existence of independent ethics review boards that assess risk and benefits of any experimental study that includes humans. Our concern is the tendency we observe to impose conditions for the approval of studies involving infants and young children that are resctritive to the point of making almost any study in this age group impossible. If this tendency were to prevail, it may pose significant obstacles to the development of our knowledge in the field of early childhood respiratory illnesses. In the case of young children who cannot give informed consent (or even assent), the demand that any study either specifically provides the involved child with a direct benefit or is associated with only minimal risk (defined in the most restrictive way) may make any invasive studies in this age group practically impossible. It is not our intention here to discuss the ethical implications of this type of requirement. We would only like to point out that, as informative as they may be, no animal study will ever be able to reproduce the specific conditions present in humans that determine the development of wheezing illnesses in early life. None of the experimental animals currently available spontaneously present the kind of lower respiratory illnesses that seem to be so common in human infants and young children. Therefore, the scientific community is faced with an extraordinary challenge: lower respiratory illnesses are the cause of significant morbidity and mortality in early life, and new approaches for prevention and treatment of this condition are badly needed. New, non-invasive methodologies will need to be developed to elucidate the immune mechanisms present in these conditions. Some hope comes from the increasing availability of studies of exhaled gases and exhaled water-vapor condensates. Both these products may provide useful information about the immune mechanisms present in the lungs of these children and the changes that may occur in these mechanisms with time. However, we are convinced that the idea that clinical science can be conducted in a completely risk-free environment is simply not sustainable. If humans are willing to drive automobiles at high speeds with their very young children aboard in circumstances that are well known to significantly increase the likelihood of accidents and death, it is difficult to conceive why they would not be willing to submit these same children to minimal risks in studies thoroughly reviewed by knowledgeable ethics committees and performed in well-controlled environments. We are convinced that informed citizens are more often than not willing to participate in, and will allow their children to participate in, studies that improve our knowledge about severe illnesses, and that perhaps may help prevent suffering and death. Because studies of immune responses occurring during wheezing illnesses in early life may require invasive studies that put young children at minimal, albeit undeniable, risk, researchers with an interest in this area should be active participants in societal discussions about how acceptable these risks may be in relation to the common good of the society as a whole. It is true that researchers involved in these kinds of studies have a vested interest and they certainly should not be the ones making the final ethical decisions in this area. However, their role in educating both the society and ethics committees about the potential benefits that all children may obtain from these studies seems, to us, crucial. Unfortunately, often these types of decisions are made by individuals who cannot truly comprehend the burden that these diseases cause to young children in developed and, especially, underdeveloped countries.

STUDIES OF THE CLINICAL AND FUNCTIONAL EVALUATION OF THE TYPICAL WHEEZY INFANT AND PRESCHOOL CHILD

Because of the age of the child, the history has to be obtained from another observer who may well interpret noisy breathing incorrectly. Physical examination in the typical wheezy child is, at best, only a very poor guide to the severity of the condition and may well be normal between attacks. Lung function tests for infants and young children are only available in specialized centers mainly concerned with research and so, at the present time, there is very little that can be done to objectively evaluate the severity of the condition or its response to treatment. This partly explains the lack of an evidence-based consensus on how to manage the typical wheezy infant. What is needed are studies aimed to provide the clinician with appropriate tools for the evaluation of the severity of the problem. These might include some or all of the following.

Studies to establish which clinical criteria can be used to evaluate the various types of typical wheezing in infancy and early childhood in order to standardize patient selection and evaluation for clinical trials

These studies should concentrate on obtaining the history using standardized question-naires, taking full account of the family history and environmental exposure to viruses, allergens and sources of endotoxin, and objectively evaluating the atopic status of the child. Physical examination can be improved by recording respiratory rate, heart rate and oxygen saturation, along with a standardized evaluation of distress and wheeze severity. There are already some studies which have objectively measured the intensity of wheeze by acoustic techniques and this should be further explored in order to refine clinical evaluation. Children should be evaluated periodically using these clinical crite-ria in an attempt to document the natural history of wheezing in infancy and early childhood, and the affect of treatment in clearly defined groups such as early wheezers, atopic persistent wheezers and non-atopic persistent wheezers.

Studies to establish new techniques for measuring lung function and bronchial responsivity in infancy and early childhood

There is a real need for office or bedside methods of evaluating the severity of the problem in very young child. While it is true than many preschool children can be induced by various games to perform simple spirometry, this is time consuming and hardly practical on an everyday basis. Infants cannot be expected to cooperate in any way with tests of lung function and so what is really needed are methods which demand nothing from the child or just passive cooperation. Pulse oximetry is a good example of this type of test but is of limited value since most wheezy infants and preschool children are not significantly desaturated. The objective measurement of wheeze intensity using an electronic stethoscope and appropriate computer software certainly deserves further exploration as this, like oximetry, is totally non-invasive and may reflect the severity of the obstruction. Work should continue to simplify the measurement of lung function in the laboratory by the various existing techniques to make them more user-friendly and applicable to a larger number of children. New approaches to the evaluation of airway inflammation, such as the measurement of exhaled nitric oxide, need to be explored as surrogate markers in wheezy infants and young children.

Studies to evaluate the clinical use of tests for measuring lung function and bronchial responsivity in infancy and early childhood

The fact that there are infants and young children who wheeze, and the fact that we do have tests which can measure lung function, does not mean that these tests provide clinically meaningful information nor that they should be widely used to evaluate the children. There is an almost total lack of information as to the clinical use of lung function testing in infants and young children, which needs to be addressed by carefully designed studies. These would probably need to be controlled, parallel-group prospective studies in which management in one group was controlled by the results of lung function tests, while in the other group the tests were performed but the results were not used to control management. Another question that needs to be addressed is the relative clinical value of different types of lung function test in this age group. Do measurements related to lung mechanics add anything to the measurements of saturation or possibly wheeze, and do more complicated tests of lung function add anything to such simple tests as the measurement of forced expiratory flow?

Studies to evaluate the basic mechanisms underlying bronchial hyperresponsivity in evaluating the various types of typical wheezing in infancy and early childhood

Asthmatic children wheeze because they have airways which narrow more readily than those of non-asthmatics to various stimuli, some of which such as exercise and the inhalation of adenosine 5'-monophosphate (AMP) are highly specific for asthma and not effective in other types of chronic lung disease of childhood. Given the uncertainty as to the pathophysiologic mechanisms at work in infants with transient early wheezing and young children with atopic or non-atopic wheezing, it would be highly desirable to perform bronchial challenges with different provoking agents in well-defined groups of children. While the auscultatory method of detecting wheeze in response to a provocation challenge (PCwheeze method) is quite suitable for the preschool child, it could be made far more objective by the automatic detection and quantification of wheeze. There is little experience with this technique, or indeed with other methods of bronchial challenge in infants, and it would be very useful to develop such methods so that studies of bronchial responsivity could be performed in the very young wheezy child.

STUDIES OF THE PREVENTION AND TREATMENT OF THE TYPICAL WHEEZY INFANT AND PRESCHOOL CHILD

Because of the lack of objective clinical and functional methods to evaluate the severity of the illness in the wheezy infant and preschool child there is also very little reliable information on the response of these children to treatment. This has been complicated by failure to appreciate that not all wheezing in this age group is the same and there exist different types of wheezy child, such as those with early transient wheezing, atopic and non-atopic wheezing. Lumping these different types of wheezy child together may well have masked important differences in the response to treatment. What is needed are studies aimed to test the efficacy of different treatment algorithms using objective means. These might include some or all of the following.

Studies to evaluate the clinical efficacy of different medications in the management of the various types of typical wheezing in infancy and early childhood

Using simple clinical criteria for classifying the children, and appropriate clinical and objective methods for following progress, controlled studies could be performed to evaluate the short-term effect of treatment with reliever (bronchodilator) and preventer (anti-inflammatory) medications. It is pertinent to know the effect of these medications on transient, atopic and non-atopic wheezing of infancy and during the preschool years. It is also important to determine whether or not there is a maturing effect with age on the response of children in the different groups of wheezy infant. Such studies should also determine the most effective short-term treatment for the management of a wheezing attack.

Studies to evaluate the most appropriate treatment algorithms for the management of the various types of typical wheezing in infancy and early childhood

Some of the important outstanding questions include whether or not preventative treatment can effectively reduce the number of recurrent episodes of wheeze, whether it can prevent continuation of wheezing into later childhood and at what stage should preventive treatment be instituted. These studies will require the longer term prospective follow-up of infants and children using objective criteria as far as possible. Because there is practically no reliable information on these problems to date, the data collected from properly controlled studies would be of use in constructing management guidelines for the wheezy infant and preschool child.

Studies of effects of anti-inflammatory therapy on the long-term outcome of wheezing in infants and young children

A widely held concept in the treatment of recurrent airway obstruction in childhood is that early initiation of therapy in some way may change the natural course of the disease process. Specifically, many pediatricians and researchers strongly believe that anti-inflammatory therapy may somehow influence the disease development process in the airways and, by this mechanism, prevent the development of symptoms later in life. Unfortunately, as we have pointed out elsewhere, this concept is supported by scanty and usually retrospective data. Such studies could be performed in parallel to those described above or could stand independently. It would be necessary for such studies to be targeted toward different forms of wheezing in early life and they should also be based on a capacity to select those subjects at the highest risk of continued wheezing later in life. For this reason, coordinating long-term epidemiologic studies on the development of genetic and clinical markers of outcome and studies in which medications are tested for the prevention of long-term sequelae of respiratory illnesses in early life would be desirable.

Index

Figures in italics indicate *tables* and *figures*.